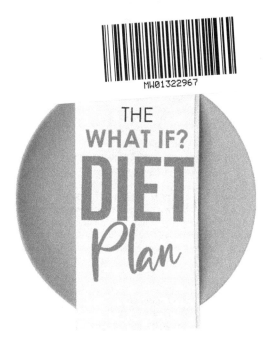

Transform your body and mind
through intermittent fasting

ALEXIS CANO

Copyright © 2020
Alexis Cano
THE WHAT IF? DIET PLAN
Transform your body and mind through intermittent fasting
All rights reserved.

No part of this publication may be reproduced, distributed, or transmitted in any form or by any means, including photocopying, recording, or other electronic or mechanical methods, without the prior written permission of the publisher, except in the case of brief quotations embodied in critical reviews and certain other non-commercial uses permitted by copyright law.

Alexis Cano

Printed in the United States of America
First Printing 2020
First Edition 2020

10 9 8 7 6 5 4 3 2 1

Alexis Cano has no responsibility for the persistence or accuracy of URLs for external or third-party Internet. Websites referred to in this publication and does not guarantee that any content on such Websites is, or will remain, accurate or appropriate.

Designations used by companies to distinguish their products are often claimed as trademarks. All brand names and product names used in this book and on its cover are tradenames, service marks, trademarks and registered trademarks of their respective owners. The publishers and the book are not associated with any product or vendor mentioned in this book. None of the companies referenced within book have endorsed the book.

ACKNOWLEDGMENTS

First and foremost, I want to thank my incredible husband for always checking-in on me and encouraging me to "believe in possibility." From the day we met, you have always seen the value in my endeavors, even when I could not. You are the kindest, most devoted father and husband, and you never cease to amaze me with your capacity to love and care for your family.

Thank you to my mother who inspires me daily to overcome life's obstacles and who taught me the value of reading and writing at an early age. You are a life-long educator who naturally instills a love of learning in your students and selflessly cares for the well-being of others over your own.

I also want to thank all my friends and family for continuously motivating me to share my message with the world and for not allowing me to give up on writing this book. I am endlessly amazed by the love and support I receive from you all!

A special thank you goes out to my dearest friend, Angelica Garza. You were taken from this world too soon, yet your spirit lives on and reminds us to live our lives to the fullest. Your imagination and creativity always bewildered me and continues to inspire me to this day. I know you are watching over us my friend, and I thank you for being our guardian angel.

REVIEWS FROM REAL WOMEN

This book is a must-read for health and wellness – not just physical attributes, but mental as well. Alexis shares her personal journey with you and encourages you to develop your own personalized plan that works for you and your family. Her sensible, real-world perspective is warm, friendly and relatable.

- Monica Castañeda, Miami, FL

I thoroughly enjoyed reading this book! It forced me to challenge my beliefs and it's wonderful how I could relate with so many things that Alexis shared… I highly recommend this book.

- Jyoti Sandhu, New Delhi, India

Through personal experience, Alexis shares her doubts and difficulties during her weight loss journey, and the solutions she discovered. Her book is very encouraging, helpful, and witty without over doing it. She also provides you with evidence-based information without overwhelming you. If you have been trying to lose weight and stay healthy, you must read this book!

- Shu-Chuan (Candace) H., Texas

WOW! A lot of what the author wrote resonated with me as I have been struggling with weight & food issues for years. Like her, I've also searched for anything that would or could help. Alexis brings out a lot of the issues that overweight people deal with during their struggles with weight and makes you feel that you are not alone.

- Barbara Simpson, Victoria, Australia

Check out www.thewhatifdietplan.com for my free ***What IF? Mindshift*** worksheet that you can use to take your "What IF?" questions to the next level! This worksheet provides you with the exact method I used to overcome my personal obstacles and take the action needed to reach my goals.

You can also find photos of me taken throughout my weight loss journey and follow my blog for more insights that I discovered along the way. I hope to see you there soon!

TABLE OF CONTENTS

PROLOGUE 1
   The Fine Print... Boring, But Necessary 4
WHAT IS THE WHAT IF DIET PLAN? 6
MY PERSONAL HISTORY WITH FOOD, WEIGHT LOSS, AND IF 8
      IF-ing in Error 8
      What's Your Secret? 13
      Breakfast + Lunch + Dinner = Freshman 15 15
      The Atkins Diet—The Answers to My Prayers... but Not My Social Life 17
      Round 2 of IF-ing in Error—What if I Have an Eating Disorder? 20
      The Carbohydrate Addicts Diet—OMG, I'm an Addict! 23
      Pregnancy to the Rescue! 25
      Portion Control to the *Max*! 26
      The Blame Game—One Man and a Baby 28
      My 4-Hour Body Couldn't Wait for Cheat Day 29
      I Want to *Want* to Lose Weight... 31
      A New Year, a New Me, but Not How I Expected It 33
WHAT IF? 35
THE SCIENCE BEHIND THE MAGIC 37
THE POWER OF HORMONES 41

  Why Restricting Calories Doesn't Work 41

  The Hunger Hormone Games.. 44

  Insulin 45

  Leptin 46

  Ghrelin 48

MIND OVER BODY 50

  Phase 1: Push It Back, Then Bring It In 50

  Now, Bring It In 55

  Trust the Plan, Not the Scale 56

  Phase 2: Shrink Your Eating Window 61

  "So When Do You Eat?" 66

  Phase 3: Watch Yourself 68

PRACTICE MAKES ~~PERFECT~~ POSSIBLE 72

WEIGHT LOSS IS A SIDE EFFECT 75

  Superhuman Energy 75

  Reduced Hunger and Mental Chatter About Food 77

  Improved Cognitive Function 80

  Autophagy 81

  Weight Loss 82

FINE-TUNE YOUR FASTING 85

  Stick to Unflavored Water, Coffee, or Tea 85

  Water, Water Everywhere... But All I Want is Diet Soda! .. 86

> What Science Says About Drinking Water 87
>
> What Science Says about Diet Soda 90
>
> Be Prepa-a-a-ared! 93
>
> Feeling Hungry? Take a Nap! 96
>
> A Full Day of Fasting 100

AFTERWORD **104**

REFERENCES **109**

PROLOGUE

What IF you could lose weight without counting calories or setting foot in a gym?

What IF you could stop food cravings, while still eating all your favorite foods?

What IF you could heal your body naturally, without cutting out entire food groups from your diet?

What IF you could live the rest of your life *never having to worry about food ever again*?

OK, I'm aware of how gimmicky this all sounds, but it is absolutely true. And quite honestly, I could go on... I haven't even mentioned the benefits of having consistent energy and mental clarity throughout the day. So, how is all this possible? Well, not necessarily by changing what you eat, but when you eat. Yes, I am referring to the popular practice of intermittent fasting, also known as IF. Many people, myself included, have heard of IF for weight loss but brush it off as a fad. Other people, myself included, may have also tried IF at some point and failed miserably because it was too hard and unrealistic.

Believe me, I get it. The thought of going more than three hours without food used to sound dreadful! By ten o'clock in the morning, my stomach would be growling and begging me for a snack. If I pushed through and made it to lunch without a snack,

I'd be "hangry" until I shoved something edible in my mouth. After lunch, I'd feel heavy, but in a much better mood... that is until three o'clock, when I needed another snack or caffeinated drink to get me through the afternoon slump. That would conveniently hold me until dinner with the family around six o'clock. But by nine or ten, I'd need another light snack, maybe some fruit and a glass of wine, to help me relax and wind down for bed. The next day, I'd start all over again.

Wow, I am exhausted just thinking about it! About how I was such a slave to food for so many years of my life. About how much of my day was occupied by thinking about food. About how much time and energy I wasted on planning my snacks and meals for the week and counting calories! About how much money I spent buying "healthy snacks" and "pre-portioned meals" so I wouldn't go overboard when I did eat. About the anxiety I felt arguing with myself about whether I should order something "healthy" or something I really wanted to eat at a restaurant. About the confusion I felt over whether I should cut my fat or carb intake. About the guilt and shame I felt when I gave in to my hunger and ended up overeating again for the fifth time in a week.

Honestly, it doesn't just exhaust me... It makes me downright pissed off! There were so many times when I wished I just didn't have to eat regular meals, or at all—that I simply didn't have an appetite. Not because I wanted to be skinny, but because life would be so much simpler. But I couldn't live off only nutritional shakes my whole life. In fact, I couldn't live off them for one day!

PROLOGUE

I never had the "willpower" necessary to stick to any kind of strict eating plan. That's probably because I undeniably *love* food!

I love to try new foods and cook for myself and friends and family. And, of course, I *love to eat*! Who doesn't? And coming from a Hispanic family, food is a huge part of our family's culture and traditions. We barbeque and drink for *every* occasion possible. And we thoroughly enjoy eating "fattening" indulgent foods just as much as "healthy" ones. These include Mexican staples, such as tacos, tamales, fajitas, and refried beans with bacon—and don't even get me started on tortilla chips with guacamole!

Fortunately, the What IF Diet Plan has allowed me to participate in all my social occasions and eat real food with my friends and family while feeling satiated, not guilty. So, if any of this resonates with you, I encourage you to give the What IF Diet Plan a chance to work for you. Never in a thousand years did I think that I would be writing a diet book, but I am so incredibly passionate about the What IF Diet Plan and fasting, that I knew I had to do my part to get the word out. The What IF Diet Plan has changed my life completely, and I know it can change yours for the better too.

The Fine Print... Boring, But Necessary

I must start by letting you know that I am not a doctor or medical professional. I am not a nutritionist or personal trainer, or any kind of expert in the field of diet and exercise. What I am is a wife and full-time working mother of three beautiful little boys who has finally discovered a simple solution to an extremely frustrating problem for many, many people. I am also an avid researcher, lifelong learner, self-experimenter of things related to health and wellness, and a big believer in holistic health and self-care. That being said, the information provided in this book should not be taken as medical advice. Please consult and work with your physician prior to following the guidelines provided here.

Also, on a serious note, if you struggle with symptoms of disordered eating or are being treated for an eating disorder, please consult with your doctor and therapist before following the What IF Diet Plan. Although the plan does not *cause* disordered eating, it may exacerbate symptoms for those already struggling with disordered eating tendencies. The What IF Diet Plan is *not* a quick-fix or starvation diet that will make you shed pounds rapidly. In fact, it is possible to gain some weight during the first phase of the diet. If the thought of gaining a few pounds fills you with dread, then the What IF Diet Plan may not be for you.

PROLOGUE

Even though I am not a doctor or expert in nutrition, I reference many sources from medical studies, journals, and books written by doctors and experts. I highly recommend reading those books and articles when you have a chance. While reading the references is not required to utilize the What IF Diet Plan, they explain many biological processes and terminologies in better detail and more eloquently than I can. Plus, if you are anything like me, reading these resources will make you feel empowered and even more in tune with your body.

You may also feel a bit aggravated when you realize that the answers have been at our fingertips the entire time, but are often overlooked or swept under the rug. If you find yourself fuming from time to time, like I did, take comfort in knowing that it is not too late to heal yourself and overcome the struggle with food. The What IF Diet Plan can work for people of all ages, ethnicities, and lifestyles—with support from your doctor(s), of course.

WHAT IS THE WHAT IF DIET PLAN?

As stated in the prologue, the What IF Diet Plan is essentially an intermittent fasting lifestyle. This diet does not limit the type or amount of food you can eat, just the time frame in which you can eat it. It also does not require calorie counting or portion control. In fact, the What IF Diet Plan is probably like no other diet you have ever tried before.

I was hesitant to even call this a "diet" since it does not focus on restricting calories or food groups, as most conventional diets do. In contrast, the What IF Diet Plan allows you to never think or worry about food again! I sought out other terms I could use instead, such as *strategy, procedure, arrangement, routine,* but nothing else seemed to fit. The term *diet* seemed a natural fit.

So, in searching for the perfect term to describe my plan, I looked up the official definition of the word *diet* in the Merriam-Webster Dictionary and found this statement:

> *But diet was used in another sense too in the Middle and early modern English periods to mean "way of living." This is, in fact, the original meaning of diet's Greek ancestor diaita, which is derived from the verb diaitasthan, meaning "to lead one's life."*

I just about fell out of my chair when I read the definition! It turns out that the original meaning for the word *diet* was *exactly* what I was looking for to describe the What IF Diet Plan. In fact, this goes to show just how skewed our view of health and nutrition has become throughout history. I now believe that the word *diet* was never meant to convey restriction or willpower. It was simply meant to convey a *way of living* one's life, which shouldn't be an endeavor. Life should be as relaxed, fruitful, and worry free as possible. This describes the What IF Diet Plan perfectly!

That being said, the What IF Diet Plan is not a quick fix. Although it is possible to lose weight quickly on the plan, that is not my main goal for you. My ultimate goal for anyone reading this book is developing a lifelong style of eating that will free you from ever having to worry about food, while also allowing your body to naturally regulate and heal itself. So, whether your goal is to lose 100 pounds, feel more energized, have clearer skin, gain muscle, etc., the What IF Diet Plan can work for you.

MY PERSONAL HISTORY WITH FOOD, WEIGHT LOSS, AND IF

IF-ing in Error

Like many people, I discovered intermittent fasting (IF) purely by accident in my late teen years. The first occurrence was during my senior year of high school, at the age of 17. Looking back, it makes plenty of sense that my body naturally took to IF, as I had ballooned up to a size 20 and at least 230 pounds during this time. My body was constantly aching, and I was always feeling tired and bloated. At this point in my life, I wanted to lose weight, but knew nothing about nutrition or calorie counting. However, I did know the basic tenet of weight loss: eat less and move more. Although, it seems impossible to move more when you can barely find the energy to roll yourself out of bed in the morning.

One morning, I arrived at school too late to eat breakfast, which our school provided for free to all students. I was upset at myself for missing breakfast since I knew it was the "most important meal of the day." I also knew that I was going to have trouble concentrating in my morning classes and would be absolutely *starving* by lunch!

Well, it seems that this little misstep ended up being one of the most transformative days in my young life, especially in my weight-loss journey.

Turns out that I did not experience the brain fog, dizziness, or overall wretchedness that I expected from missing breakfast. I felt just fine, although my stomach was definitely growling by the time lunch rolled around. So I ate lunch as usual and went on about my day. Lunch usually consisted of pizza, Frito pie, Flamin' Hot Cheetos with cheese, or a sub sandwich—whatever was available to purchase at the school's snack bar. Since I was trying to eat "healthier" though, I made an effort to eat a piece of fruit as well. For the next few weeks, I decided to experiment and continued to purposely skip breakfast to see how my body reacted.

After a few weeks, I noticed that I was feeling lighter and more energetic in the mornings. It actually felt good to have an empty stomach and allow myself to feel "real hunger" for the first time in years. Plus, I loved the convenience of not having to rush to school to make sure I got breakfast in. I didn't own a scale at the time (yes, I know that's shocking, but I was not a very body-conscious teenager), but I could swear my clothes were fitting looser. I figured that if I was losing weight, it was probably due to eating fewer calories by skipping breakfast. It made perfect sense: eat less + move more = weight loss.

One day, I had to cram for a biology exam that I had forgotten about (i.e., procrastinated on) until the day it was scheduled.

Fortunately, it was my last class of the day, so I figured I could study during lunch. The only problem was, no food or drinks were allowed in the library. I was already used to skipping breakfast, but there was no way that I could survive skipping lunch. I figured I could always buy a snack and scarf it down between classes and studying for this exam was priority. So, I reluctantly passed my friends' lunch table and hunkered down in the school library for an hour to study.

I wish I could say that I was super focused and that studying was a breeze, but not even IF has that power! As usual, I was unorganized and probably did a horrible job of cramming in as much information as I could so I could pass my test. Although I love to read and learn new things, school was never my forte. My stomach was also growling the entire time, which probably didn't help my concentration. In any case, I pushed through, attended the rest of my classes, and took my biology exam. I honestly don't even remember if I passed it or not.

However, I *do* remember noticing that my hunger had passed after a while. Even though I was *starving* during lunch, my stomach had stopped growling, and I didn't feel like passing out, like I thought I would. That being said, I knew it was dangerous to skip too many meals. I saw that episode of *Full House* where D.J. faints from starving herself to try to lose weight. The last thing I wanted was for my big butt to pass out in class in front of all my friends and classmates. I would be mortified!

So, ignoring my body's cues, I grabbed something quick from the snack bar and scarfed it down in between classes as I had originally planned. Once I got home, I ate dinner as usual. However, over the next few weeks, I noticed times that I wasn't hungry when lunch rolled around. Sometimes I was surprised that it was lunch already, because I was so focused on my school work. I wasn't looking at the clock every five minutes or counting down until lunch like I used to.

One day I decided to follow my body's cues. I found it awkward to sit in the cafeteria with my friends and *not* eat, so I made some excuse that I had to study, or read, or whatever, and made my way to the library instead. Once there, I felt strange. What would I do with myself during lunch if I wasn't going to eat?

Fortunately, I was an avid reader and artist, so I was able to find several books that I wanted to read, and on the days I didn't feel like reading, I would sketch. At first, this time felt very strange, and almost shameful. I was supposed to be in the cafeteria eating with my friends, but I felt so out of place *not eating* when I was *not hungry* that I chose to hide out in the library instead. Shame! Shame! Shame!

Cue Cerci from Game of Thrones walking through the town square naked. OK, that's a bit dramatic, but it's how I felt at the time.

After a couple of weeks, my friends started asking me why I was spending so much time in the library and what exactly was I doing. I admitted that I really wasn't studying or doing anything important, I just wasn't hungry during lunch and found it awkward sitting in the cafeteria not eating while everyone else was eating. Plus, I didn't want to influence their decisions as to whether they should eat or not.

Like good friends should, they simply laughed when they heard my reason for going to the library during lunch and even offered to join me. When I told them that I didn't want them to not eat on my account, they enlightened me to the fact that everyone snuck food into the library, so it really wasn't a big deal. They would much rather join me in the back of the library and eat a contraband sacked lunch than a crappy Frito pie from the cafeteria snack bar. Furthermore, my decision to eat or not eat was my own, and they wouldn't infringe on my decision unless they felt it that was affecting me negatively, which they didn't. Wow, did I feel stupid for not giving my friends enough credit!

And so this continued for the remainder of my senior year. I spent my lunch hour in the library most days, and my closest group of friends usually joined me, unless they had other commitments or felt like eating in the cafeteria that day.

And my decisions to eat or not eat lunch weren't impacting anyone in a negative way, as I feared they would.

What's Your Secret?

Around this time, my peers really started noticing and complimenting me on my weight loss. Classmates stopped me in the hallways to ask how much weight I'd lost and what I was doing. I never knew what to say because I genuinely didn't know how much weight I'd lost, and I didn't feel like I was "doing" anything to lose weight. A few times I stammered, "Um... not eating," but that never felt right. Looking back, I wish I'd said, "Listening to my body's natural hunger cues and not eating just because the clock says it's time to eat," but it never came out so articulately. Does it ever?

The term *intermittent fasting* did not exist during this time in the late '90s—at least not to my knowledge. The closest terms I could think of to describe what I was doing were *dieting* or *starving myself*, neither of which were accurate. I didn't feel like I was "dieting" since I really wasn't monitoring my food intake or counting fat grams, calories, or points. And I definitely wasn't "starving myself" because I still ate plenty of food. I just wasn't eating it throughout my entire waking day, like I used to.

Another thing I noticed around this time was that my tastes and food cravings were changing. Fast food was not tasting nearly as tasty as before. Instead, it started tasting fake. Pizza was way too salty, and packaged snack cakes tasted all "chemically." I used to love eating junk food snacks after school. In fact, I used to stop at the closest fast food joint and order a couple of double meat cheeseburgers, or tater tots with chili and cheese, or onion rings, or fried chicken sandwiches, or a milkshake *before* I got home and ate dinner.

However, after a few weeks of skipping breakfast and lunch, I found that those foods weren't hitting the spot for me anymore. I started craving home-cooked meals instead. My grandmother lived with us, which is common in Mexican culture, and she cooked for the family every night. In the past, I had found her cooking bland and boring, but I noticed that after fasting throughout the day, her home-cooked meals were unbelievably satisfying. And it was not because I was so hungry that anything would have tasted good; otherwise, fast food should have tasted twice as good. On the rare occasions that she didn't cook, I began experimenting with my own recipes. I would make homemade lentils and rice, chicken noodle soup, or a giant chef salad with freshly fried bacon, boiled eggs, sharp cheddar cheese, and thick creamy ranch dressing. Yum!

Before I knew it, prom was coming up. I was by no means "skinny," but I for sure wasn't 230 pounds any longer.

It had been at least three months since I started IF-ing in error, and I'd already had to purchase a whole new wardrobe. But I still had no idea how much weight I'd lost. Out of pure curiosity, I snuck into the locker room at school to weigh myself: 185 pounds… OMG. Although I was still technically overweight for my 5'6" frame, I was shocked to see that I had lost 45 pounds in those few months—without even trying. I wasn't slaving away at the gym or counting calories or Weight Watchers points; I was just *not eating* when I was *not hungry*.

Seeing my newfound weight loss on the scale felt better than I ever imagined! I always knew that I was overweight, but it never felt like something that I could control, so I never really cared about it. Now that I had tangible evidence that I could control my weight, and with such little effort on my part, what else was I capable of? That night I went home and did my first round of calisthenics on the floor of my bedroom while Conan O'Brian played in the background. If I could lose weight, maybe I could also firm up my thighs? My butt? My arms? My abs? Could I get abs? Was that also a possibility? Of course it was! It's amazing how losing 45 pounds can change one's outlook on life.

Breakfast + Lunch + Dinner = Freshman 15

By the time I got to college, I'd lost a bit more weight throughout the rest of my senior year and the summer break. I weighed a comfortable 160 pounds and fit into size 8 jeans. The only problem was, I knew I wouldn't be able to continue skipping meals like I was so used to. First of all, my doting mother had purchased a meal plan along with my dorm room, which included three meals a day and an a-la-carte option, in case I wanted a snack or dessert whenever. Second, I lived in the on-campus dorms and was attached at the hip with my awesome new roommate, who always ate three square meals a day and was perfectly svelte! Plus, I was ashamed about skipping meals in high school. I felt that skipping meals was not healthy, and saw college life as an opportunity to get my body back in sync with a "normal" eating regimen.

So, every morning before our eight o'clock class, I'd roll myself out of bed and drag myself to the cafeteria to eat an oh-so-healthy breakfast of oatmeal with a splash of milk, artificial sweetener, cinnamon, and some fruit. I never really enjoyed breakfast, but I chalked it up to me not being a morning person. Then after our morning classes, we'd head back to the cafeteria for lunch, and I usually ended up eating much more than intended to because there were so many options to choose from. I would get a giant salad, because I knew it was good for me, and a sandwich packed with veggies to fill me up, then a burger or other entrée, of which I would take only a couple of bites just to taste. Then I would finish my meal off with a piece of fruit for dessert.

After our evening study groups, we'd head back to the cafeteria for dinner, at which point I had a voracious appetite! I was so tired and hungry that I would just skip the salad, figuring I'd already taken care of that requirement at lunch, and eat whatever entrée was on special that night. And what better way to finish off a long day of schoolwork, studying, and church activities than with a piece of cake, cookies, or an ice cream cone? And the next day, I'd do it *all… over… again*.

As you can imagine, my weight flew back up. I gained about 15-20 pounds within the first semester. My clothes got tighter, and my confidence diminished. Surprisingly, the worst part was not gaining weight; it was the loss of control over my eating habits. Breakfast was easy because I was never hungry in the morning. I simply ate oatmeal, fruit, or an egg white omelet because I knew it was good for me, and it would "rev my metabolism" to burn more fat. At lunch, I was never really *hungry* either, but for some reason found it harder to limit myself to healthier food options like I did at breakfast. By the time dinner rolled around, all bets were off!

I'd lost all self-control by this point in the day and ate everything with reckless abandon. Afterward, I'd feel guilty and promise myself that the next day would be different.

The Atkins Diet—The Answers to My Prayers... but Not My Social Life

After the first year of college, I became obsessed with food, nutrition, and controlling my weight. On the weekends, I'd visit our local second-hand book store and research as much as I could about nutrition, exercise, and anything that would make it easier to maintain my weight without having to "starve" myself like I had in high school. I look back, though, and realize I never felt like I had done that in high school. In fact, I was not obsessed with food like I was in college. I actually felt more in tune with my body then. I ate when I was hungry and didn't eat when I wasn't. It was so simple. But everyone knew that skipping meals was bad and not normal. I certainly didn't want to be judged or labeled as having an eating disorder. And quite honestly, at that point, I couldn't skip a meal if I wanted to. My body was so used to having several meals and snacks a day, it would have been torture to try.

Thus, I kept returning to the second-hand bookstore, where I found *The Volumetrics Diet Plan*. The plan was to fill up on low-calorie foods, such as soups, fruits, and veggies, so you're not hungry or tempted to eat junk. This plan worked well for keeping my weight down, but I still didn't feel like I had control over my eating. I would eat massive portions of these foods, then feel bloated and sick afterward.

Then one day, I stumbled onto the book that I thought would change my life—an original version of *Dr. Atkins' Diet Revolution*. It was old and unassuming, but since a doctor wrote it, the plan seemed legit. I purchased the book and dove in to see what it was all about. I was in awe of what this doctor claimed: You could lose weight by eating nothing but meat, cheese, bacon, and butter. Apparently, one of his patients ate 5,000 calories a day and still lost weight. And, it was virtually impossible to overeat meat and fat. Why hadn't I known about this before?

I felt like I had unearthed a priceless hidden gem. For the past year, I had been avoiding red meat, real bacon, egg yolks, and oil like the plague. Yet this doctor was touting that's what I should've been eating instead? It was the answer to my dietary prayers because I *loved* meat, cheese, bacon, and butter! Of course, I also liked fruit, potatoes, and bread, but I was willing to give them up if it meant freedom from dieting and worrying about food.

The only problem was, I was living in the college dorm with a full meal plan, and a group of friends who would have thought me insane if I told them I was going to try an all meat diet. Despite that, I decided to give it a shot. For breakfast I ate eggs with spinach, cheese, and bacon. For lunch, I ate a giant chef salad with creamy ranch dressing, or a bunless sandwich or cheeseburger if I felt brave. For dinner, I'd just try my best to eat whatever meat was on the menu that night. When I got hungry in between meals, I would eat boiled eggs or pork rinds for a snack. My poor roommate put up with so many weird smells during that time! For the most part though, following the Atkins diet worked well... for about two weeks.

Then I found myself craving everyday foods that I once took for granted. I would have killed for one bite of an apple! Plus, I found myself becoming less and less social simply because I didn't want people watching me eat my plate of greasy meat. Although low carb and keto are common now, they were not so popular in the early 2000s. There was no such thing as low-carb or gluten-free options back then, especially in the rural college town I lived in. Everyone ate meat and potatoes, as well as rice and beans, and you couldn't have one without the other.

The final straw for the Atkins Diet was when I decided to start cooking my own food in the dorm kitchen so I could plan my meals and not have to worry about the sparse low-carb fare from the dining hall. Of course, this meant I was spending hours on Sundays cooking in the shared kitchen, packing everything in Tupperware containers, and then stuffing them in the mini fridge in our room. It also meant that while my friends went to the dining hall to eat, I would make my way back to my dorm room, microwave my food, and sit and eat the most depressing, greasy meals ever.

On top of that, I found I was still stuffing my face and thinking about food constantly. I didn't gain any weight, but I felt worse about myself and food than I ever felt before. So I decided to ditch the Atkins Diet and continue my search for the perfect diet plan.

Fortunately, I was quite active during my college years. I took swimming and weight-training courses, and ran several miles a day to keep in shape. I also started walking after each meal because I read somewhere that it aided digestion. Sure, I was still eating monster-sized portions, but I was so active that I could pretty much eat whatever I wanted and still keep my weight down. In fact, it became like a game of "Let's see how much Alexis is going to eat today." I had my social life back and could eat with reckless abandon, as long as I continued to lift weights and run laps like a mad woman. Sounded like a good, solid plan to me.

Round 2 of IF-ing in Error—What if I Have an Eating Disorder?

Fast-forward a few of years to my early 20s. I was out of college and held a managerial position at a fast food restaurant, (go figure!) I worked the breakfast/lunch shift, so my hours were from 6 a.m. to 4 p.m. As you can imagine, it was a struggle waking up at 5 a.m. to make and eat breakfast at home and get to work on time. And once I got to work, I was constantly on the go until about 2 p.m., just after the lunch rush.

One morning, I didn't feel like waking up at dawn to make breakfast. I figured I'd sleep in and grab something to eat at work. I hit the snooze button a few times, then rolled out of bed to get dressed and head to work. As soon as I walked in, the breakfast crowd slammed us, so I grabbed a cup of coffee and knew I'd have to wait to eat breakfast until after the rush. By 8 a.m., I was *hungry*! I felt like I was going to pass out if I didn't get something in me soon, but the breakfast rush was at its peak, and I told myself that I'd have to wait.

Once the rush passed, I quickly made a breakfast sandwich for myself. To my surprise though, my intense hunger and fatigue had passed as well. I was still hungry, but not ravenous like I'd been an hour before. I found this interesting and pondered it while I enjoyed my food. I thought back to high school when I used to skip breakfast and lunch, and eat only dinner, and wondered if I should try that again.

As soon as the thought entered my mind, though, I slapped myself mentally as if I were about to touch something forbidden. I told myself that skipping meals was *not* good. Skipping meals would wreak havoc on my body and slow my metabolism. My body needed consistent nourishment throughout the day, and depriving it of sustenance was cruel and unhealthy.

Despite this mental conflict, I found myself naturally pushing my breakfast back further and further into the day. It was so convenient not making breakfast in the mornings, or taking a 30-minute break to scarf down food that I couldn't enjoy. Eventually, my energy levels increased. I flitted around the restaurant like a hummingbird on steroids cooking, taking inventory, unloading the truck, counting money, and doing whatever needed to get done—and with energy to spare. After work, I'd go home and cook or go out and eat whatever I felt like enjoying that day. It was great!

However, I still felt very conflicted about this lifestyle. My co-workers would pick on me for not eating, which didn't bother me. I would simply tell them that I wasn't hungry and be done with it. What did bother me was when my family members commented on my eating patterns and shrinking frame. Although I was not trying to lose weight, I had indeed lost several pounds in the year after I left college. I weighed between 130 and 135 pounds, which was perfectly healthy for my 5'6" frame, but my Hispanic family constantly commented that I wasn't eating enough and was way too skinny.

Although I didn't feel too skinny or weak or frail, I grew a little concerned myself. I *knew* I should be eating three to five times a day for optimal health, so why didn't I just do that? I knew why. Because when I did eat small meals throughout the day, I would eventually lose control and overeat. And not just once, or on special occasions, but every day! I hated that feeling of being out of control with my eating. It was so much easier to just eat something I really enjoyed at the end of the day, rather than try to control my eating throughout the entire day. I started thinking, Do I have an eating disorder? Why can't I just eat like a normal human being?

The Carbohydrate Addicts Diet—OMG, I'm an Addict!

In my continued quest for the perfect diet plan, I stumbled upon *The Carbohydrate Addict's Diet: The Lifelong Solution to Yo-Yo Dieting*. Unlike *Dr. Atkins' Diet Revolution*, this book spoke to me. I didn't think I was a "carbohydrate addict," but I clearly saw myself as a yo-yo dieter with my tendency to skip meals.

I learned I was most likely addicted to carbohydrates due to their effects on insulin and blood sugar. To avoid spikes in both of those, all I had to do was eat two small low-carb meals consisting of lean meat and veggies per day, and then one reward meal of anything I wanted—but it had to be consumed within an hour. Doing so would keep insulin spikes to a minimum, blood sugar steady, and my metabolism burning fat for fuel. And since I could eat a reward meal once per day, I should not feel deprived. It sounded like a win!

So I meal prepped chicken breasts and broccoli, or pork tenderloin with asparagus, or salmon and green beans to eat for breakfast and lunch each day. I decided to have my one-hour reward meal at dinner. As you can imagine, eating warmed-up meat and veggies for breakfast was *not* fun. Breakfast was hard enough for me to eat when it was something I enjoyed, such as bacon and eggs, but it had become a total gag-fest. But I knew it would rev up my metabolism and keep my body nourished throughout the day. I reminded myself that I would later have my reward meal and could eat whatever I wanted.

So for dinner, I would have whatever entrée I felt like eating, plus some fruit, and maybe some dessert. The only problem was that it all had to be eaten within an hour. The doctors who wrote the book clearly stated that the reward meal should not be an all-you-can-eat smorgasbord of sweets and junk food. Even though you could eat whatever you wanted, the aim was not to stuff your face with everything you can cram in there. Unfortunately, that was usually my result.

I would eat dinner and some fruit for dessert, but then I'd also want to fit in the small bag of chips that was left over from lunch. Oh, and that piece of cake that I saved from a friend's party. Before I knew it, I was stuffing my face with all the "reward food" I could eat because I knew I had only an hour to eat it. When going out to eat with my friends, I would nibble on appetizers and sip drinks, then eat the main course, but would feel defeated when the reward hour passed, and I was still drinking and sharing dessert with them.

Before I knew it, I became obsessed with food again! What could I eat for my two low-carb meals? What could/should I eat for my reward meal? If I was having lunch with a friend, that meant I'd need to make that my reward meal and restrict myself to a low-carb pre-portioned meal at night, which I hated. I enjoyed eating dinner and snacking with my boyfriend after a long day at work, and did not want to count calories or carbs when I was trying to relax. Although my boyfriend always supported my latest diet scheme, he had no desire in joining me or restricting his meals in any way.

Pregnancy to the Rescue!

You don't hear that every day, but that is truly how I felt about my pregnancy. At 24 years old, I became pregnant with my first son, and I was now eating for two and had more to be concerned about than my weight. I had to nourish my baby with a variety of fruits, veggies, fats, proteins, and vitamins and minerals. No more counting calories or carbs for me! Instead of restricting my food choices, I expanded my food choices... as well as my intake.

In fact, I gained 70 pounds throughout that pregnancy. Yikes! I ate a very healthy diet of spinach, blueberries, walnuts, salmon, yogurt, etc. But I also ate a lot of tortilla chips with guacamole, Margherita pizza, steak and potatoes, bagels and cream cheese, etc. Much like when I was IF-ing in error, I felt free from the worry of what and when to eat. I simply ate when I felt like eating. Perhaps I wasn't always eating because I was truly hungry, but I ate what I wanted when I wanted and did not feel guilty about it, which was great!

Despite my massive weight gain, my first pregnancy was a dream. I had lots of energy and was always in a good mood. My skin was clear and glowing, and my hair was thick and shiny. It's a good thing too, because I ended up carrying my son past full term and gave birth at 42 weeks on the dot. I was in labor for almost 24 hours, but bounced back quickly after giving birth. I also produced plenty of breast milk and was fortunate to breastfeed exclusively for six months. I felt like much of this was due to having a varied, well-balanced diet and letting go of the worry I always had about food.

Portion Control to the *Max*!

Of course, once I had given birth to my son, it was time to get back in the groove and ditch the dreaded baby weight. Since I was still breastfeeding, I knew I could not do anything drastic, like skip meals or cut out whole food groups. I decided that meal prepping and pre-portioning my meals was the way to go. I could portion my meals and snacks to make sure that I had enough nutrition to support my milk supply and still lose the excess weight.

I bought a whole new set of Tupperware and lots of healthy snacks, such as nuts, seeds, fiber cereal, protein bars, frozen fruit, and yogurt. I weighed and measured everything so I had three small meals and three snacks per day. It was a perfect no-fail plan because of how structured it was. I would eat one of my pre-portioned meals or snacks every two to three hours so I would never be hungry, and my body would have a steady stream of nourishment for breastmilk production. At the time, I worked in a nice, fast-paced office setting with co-workers who were also very much into exercise and nutrition, so following my plan during the workday was a breeze.

However, following this plan at home in the evenings and on weekends was maddening! For the first six months of our son's life, my husband stayed home with him, which I was extremely grateful for. However, that meant I was on baby duty as soon as I walked in the door. I was also pumping milk every two to three hours, so between caring for the baby and pumping, keeping track of my scheduled meals and snacks was the last thing on my mind. Plus, who wants to eat pre-portioned meals after a long day at work?

My husband is an excellent cook and had dinner ready every evening when I got home from work. One of my favorites was baked chicken with mashed potatoes, yeast rolls, and homemade gravy. A couple of nights a week, he'd bake an apple or cherry pie with crumb topping for dessert, which I could never resist taking a few bites of. Although I was not eating horribly during this time, I still felt guilty for not sticking to my pre-portioned meals and snacks and giving in to eating real food. Sometimes I would eat a healthy snack in the car on my way home so I wouldn't be hungry at dinner. Of course, that never worked. In fact, I often felt even hungrier after eating the stupid snack! I felt like I just couldn't win.

The Blame Game—One Man and a Baby

I ended up losing the baby weight after about nine months. I continued to eat my small pre-portioned meals while avoiding my husband's home cooking, and ran two or three miles a day on our home treadmill. It was not fun running, or doing any physical activity, when my breasts were producing milk, but I was finally able to squeeze into my size 6 pants again, which felt worth it at the time.

Almost simultaneously, I was plagued with the baby blues *big* time. I had been laid off from my cushy job in the big city, and my husband and I decided to move back to his small hometown to be closer to family. While I tried my hardest to see the silver lining, I was definitely depressed and grew very bitter toward my husband and even my son, (although I did my best to hide it from him).

Like many women do, I masked my feelings of depression and anxiety as best I could by focusing *even more* on food and exercise. Secretly, I resented and blamed my husband for my food and body issues. There was a constant loop of blame and negativity playing through my head saying:

If he would just support me by not keeping junk food in the house, it wouldn't be so hard for me to lose weight!

If he hadn't gotten me pregnant, I wouldn't even have to lose this stupid weight in the first place!

If he hadn't moved our family to this rinky-dink little town with no healthy eating options or a decent place to exercise, I would have lost this weight months ago!

And on and on it went.

Looking back, I know I didn't really believe these absurd thoughts. My husband was my biggest supporter and worked extremely hard to try to make me happy—probably to a fault. But it was easier to blame him for my unhappiness and issues with food than to think there was something wrong with me, as I had in college. I was following every single healthy eating tip imaginable, but still always felt hungry. I was eating five or six small meals a day consisting of low-fat yogurt, Fiber One cereal, plain oatmeal with cinnamon, baked fish and chicken breasts, tons of salads and veggies, omega-3 capsules, protein shakes, green tea, etc. Yet, it seemed like no matter what volume of food I was eating, I was always *hungry* for more.

My 4-Hour Body Couldn't Wait for Cheat Day

In 2010 Tim Ferriss released *The 4-Hour Body*. I thoroughly enjoyed his first book, *The 4-Hour Work Week*, and loved his concept of *Lifestyle Design*, so I was excited to see what gold nuggets Ferriss would offer in this new book. Not surprisingly, Ferriss did not fail to deliver. In *The 4-Hour Body*, he introduced the concept of the *Minimum Effective Dose*. I was *hooked*!

As a new mom with more than just myself to think about, this concept was exactly what I was looking for. I no longer had time to work out for several hours a day or the budget to buy fancy, expensive protein bars and powders. According to Ferriss, I could do some squats and wall-presses, and eat very economically and drop weight *fast*. The Slow Carb Diet that he outlined in the book had only five extremely simple rules, which were much less restrictive than what I'd been trying to do. Best of all... I could eat as much as I wanted of the approved foods and indulge in a weekly cheat day, which he referred to as a "Dieters Gone Wild" day. This truly was a dieter's dream come true!

I wasted no time stocking up on eggs, lentils, spinach, and chicken to get started on my new diet plan. However, I had one problem. Ferriss insisted that people must eat "within one hour of waking" and that forgetting to do so (or skipping breakfast altogether) would result in fat-loss failure. It was also critical that each meal supplied "at least 20 grams of protein." Gag! I already didn't enjoy eating breakfast so early, but eating eggs with spinach and lentils made it so much worse. I'd drive to work feeling so bloated and nauseated from having such a full stomach. To make downing 20 grams of protein easier, I later tried chugging a small protein shake instead. Big mistake.

Despite my abhorrence to eating beans and lentils for breakfast, I followed the diet strictly throughout the week. But I never felt satiated after eating a slow-carb meal as the book described. And just like every other diet I tried, I ended up feeling stuffed, bloated, and still hungry! My saving grace was my "Dieters Gone Wild" cheat day... or so I thought.

I don't know why I thought it would be different this time around. I could barely handle a daily reward meal years before, let alone an entire cheat day! As I should have guessed, Friday nights were hard to stick to my new diet plan. I didn't want to eat meat, beans, and greens when I went out for dinner and drinks with friends. So I'd give in and eat what everyone else was eating, figuring Friday would be my cheat day. Then came Saturday, my original cheat day, when I'd feel cheated out of not having a full cheat day and end up cheating more on that day too. By Sunday, I couldn't care less about eating an early breakfast or no/low/slow carbs. I'd just have a big mug of coffee with sugar-free vanilla creamer and tell myself that I'd start again on Monday. As much as I admire Tim Ferriss, the slow-carb diet just wasn't for me.

I Want to *Want* to Lose Weight...

Fast forward eight years and two more kids later. My weight had fluctuated greatly over the years, from 150 pounds before being pregnant with my second son, to 220 pounds after giving birth to my third. Almost three years after my third son was born, my weight finally stagnated around 200 pounds. By this point, I had pretty much given up on trying to lose weight through diet and exercise. I felt like I wanted to *want* to lose weight, but I didn't feel like *trying* anymore.

I finally decided it was time to love and accept my body and eating habits as they were. Sure, I was overweight, but I felt healthy and was still pretty active. In fact, I had been walking three to five miles every day for the past two years. There was no way I could keep that up if I wasn't healthy, right? I figured that I was in my mid-thirties and a mother of three small children. It was normal to be a bit on the heavy side, especially since I wasn't running and weight training as I had been in my 20s. Plus, my metabolism was probably wrecked from so many years of yo-yo dieting and skipping meals in my younger years. This was punishment for my dietary sins, and accepting my chubby body was my penance.

So I decided to forget about dieting and counting calories, or cutting out carbs or gluten or sugar. I strived to eat a healthy, balanced diet, but refused to restrict myself as I had done before. I also kept taking my daily walks and even joined a high-intensity interval training (HIIT) class three days a week, which I had a love/hate relationship with. I loathed all the huffing and puffing during class, and being drenched in sweat afterward; but I was impressed that I could keep up with girls who were 10 years younger than me. I also began meditating several times a week, which really helped me gain compassion for myself and focus my energy on more constructive avenues. I was still overweight and not exactly comfortable in my body but decided that I would focus on being a strong, healthy wife and mother, rather than a miserable skinny chick.

A New Year, a New Me, but Not How I Expected It

For the 2018 New Year, I continued to focus on being a happier, healthier, more passionate person. This was the first year since college that I didn't even bother trying to lose weight or making a New Year's resolution, which was quite liberating. I continued to attend my HIIT class two or three times a week; was in the second semester of my master's program; was scheduled to train at a national conference in May; and had two of my three kids in school. Life was pretty darn good... and extremely busy!

One day, I was scrolling through the Amazon Prime documentary selections and came across a documentary titled *The Science of Fasting*. I was intrigued and figured I'd give it a try. As I watched, I was shocked to hear some of the claims being made about the benefits of fasting. Doctors in other countries were using it to treat certain diseases and cancer? The negative side effects of chemotherapy were lessened in patients who fasted? And wait—fasting didn't slow the metabolism or result in extreme muscle loss?

As intriguing as the documentary was, I brushed it aside and tried to forget about it. At this point in my life, there was no way that I could fast or drink nothing but water and bone broth all day. In fact, I had heard about IF and *calorie restriction* a few years before, but failed miserably when I tried the plans that were popular at the time: *Eat Stop Eat* and the "5:2 Diet". I couldn't even last two days! I had decided that I was *not* going to put myself through another anguishing diet again. Besides, most of the people featured in *The Science of Fasting* were patients with chronic or serious illnesses who used fasting as a last resort. Not 30-something-year-old mothers who wanted to lose a few pounds. I told myself, "Girl, don't even think about it." And I listened. After watching that obscure documentary though, I started noticing the terms *fasting* and *intermittent fasting* everywhere.

Apparently, Ronda Rousey intermittent fasted during her UFC days. Even body builders and NFL players claimed to use intermittent fasting (IF) for optimal health and athletic gains. Before I could get excited about another new dieting venture though, I told myself to snap out of it. IF was just a fad that became popular with the whole paleo/caveman diet craze and would only lead to more yo-yo dieting. I had already promised myself that I was done with dieting and punishing my body by restricting food. And what could be more restrictive than fasting?

WHAT IF?

The more I tried to ignore the science behind fasting, the more drawn to it I became. I remembered in my earlier years how good I felt going all day without eating and then enjoying a fulfilling meal with family and friends. I remembered how light I felt not having a full stomach all day. I remembered how much energy I had from drinking coffee during the day, and not having to worry about what or when I would eat breakfast or lunch. I remembered how freeing it was not worrying about food or feeling hungry all the time. I remembered how effortless it was to keep my weight down without even trying. But, I also remembered how guilty I felt that I had "neglected" my body and health by skipping meals.

What if I hadn't wrecked my body in my younger years by skipping meals like I thought? *What if* eating small meals throughout the day was actually making it harder not to overeat and maintain a healthy weight? *What if* fasting could help me lose the extra weight I'd gained after having kids? *What if* fasting could be part of a busy, healthy lifestyle... even for a mother of three kids?

Then it hit me: This would be my *What IF? Diet Plan*. And *if* it worked, it would be the last diet plan I'd ever need. So I decided to start the What IF Diet Plan to see if it could work for me.

However, I decided I would only stay on this plan under three conditions:

1. It could not interfere with my family, work, or social life.

2. It had to be convenient and cost effective.

3. I would not take part in any form of exercise or physical activity that I did not enjoy.

That was it. If at any point I found that the What IF Diet Plan did not meet one of these three conditions, I would end it and move on. Thus, my pursuit of the What IF Diet Plan began.

THE SCIENCE BEHIND THE MAGIC

As mentioned in my disclaimer at the beginning of this book, I am not a medical expert. However, when I hear about something connected to health and wellness, I am an avid researcher, lifelong learner, and self-experimenter. I like to do a quick search in my phone's browser to see what pops up whenever I catch word of something that's alleged to improve health and vitality. If it's something that really sparks my interest, or that I find hard to believe, I turn to my university's online library to investigate further.

When I began researching the benefits of fasting, I was blown away by how much research had been done on the topic. I couldn't believe that these findings weren't better known in society. Numerous studies showed that IF was an effective way to lose weight and build muscle.[1-4] One study even found that fasting could reduce levels of toxic metals in the blood.[5] Still others reported that extended fasting can regenerate stem cells and reset your immune system.[6,7]

Ironically though, reading all these cool scientific studies did nothing to motivate me to start. I had several critical thoughts swirling through my head, like, *Fasting is just too hard; I'll have to try one day when I'm not busy and can give my full attention to the process*, and *Maybe I should book a fasting retreat?* In fact, reading all the research on fasting only kept me stagnant and more indecisive about actually *doing* it.

In fact, a famous British study from 2002 found that simply knowing more about a concept didn't motivate people to participate in it more.[8] In the study, 248 participants were randomly assigned to three groups. One group was asked to read the opening of a novel, then record their exercise habits for the next two weeks. The second group was asked to read "factual information about [coronary heart disease] and the benefits of exercise," then record their exercise habits for the next two weeks. The third group was given the same factual information to read, but was also asked to complete this statement:

"During the next week I will partake in at least 20 minutes of vigorous exercise on (day or days) _____ at_____ (time of day) at/or in (place) _____."

The results revealed that although the factual information significantly increased the second group's *intention* to exercise, there was no significant difference in the amount of exercise *performed* when compared to the group that read the opening of a novel. However, the statement that the third group was instructed to complete seemed to have a "dramatic effect on subsequent exercise behavior." These types of statements are known as *implementation intentions,* and they consist of creating a simple plan to explain exactly where, when, and how you will carry out an intended task.

THE SCIENCE BEHIND THE MAGIC

I provide you with this information to let you know that you can start the What IF Diet Plan now, even if you don't know (or care to know) the science behind fasting. This chapter will provide plenty of insight about hunger, fat metabolism, autophagy, etc., but it's not a prerequisite for starting your journey to improved health. So, if you're eager to get started, please feel free to skip to the section titled *Mind Over Body*. You can always come back and read the science-y stuff later, which I highly recommend.

That being said, there are a few basics about fasting and metabolism that might be helpful to know:

1. Sweetness spikes insulin (not to be confused with blood sugar) and stimulates hunger.

2. The body can use its own fat for fuel and energy, but is more efficient at burning fat for fuel once glycogen stores are depleted.

3. Fasting induces a natural process called *autophagy* that acts as a "clean-up crew" inside the body.

4. Fasting allows the body to rest and heal itself naturally.

A lot of sound science backs up the benefits of fasting that go way beyond weight loss. So, if you're a health nerd like me and interested in learning more about fat loss, insulin resistance, autophagy, etc., I highly recommend that you read an incredible book titled *The Obesity Code*, by Dr. Jason Fung. Dr. Fung has a way of explaining the biological processes of the body in simple and memorable ways. He also offers lots of free information on The Fasting Method blog and numerous YouTube videos.

Dr. Valter Longo is another great resource for finding out the science behind fasting. He is the author of *The Longevity Diet* and founder of the Create Cures Foundation. He was also featured in that obscure documentary I watched, *The Science of Fasting*, which sparked the idea for The What IF Diet Plan. Dr. Longo performed groundbreaking research and found that fasting can help the body offset the negative effects of chemotherapy and possibly improve its effectiveness in fighting cancer cells.

THE POWER OF HORMONES

Why Restricting Calories Doesn't Work

You might be thinking, if restricting calories doesn't work, why do I know so many people who have lost weight by cutting calories? Well, while it is possible for most people to lose weight by restricting the number of calories they consume, it is just as likely that they will regain the weight they've lost once they stop dieting and go back to eating "normally." This is exactly why I suggest that *restricting calories doesn't work.*

Besides, if losing weight was a matter of simply reducing our caloric intake, wouldn't we all just choose to eat 1,200 calories a day and look like swimsuit models? I know I would! The truth is that there's much more to losing fat and slimming down than the number of calories we intend to eat each day. In my case, *hunger* was a huge factor that kept me from sticking to any kind of restriction diet.

I would start my day off with good intentions, planning to eat only 1,500 calories throughout the day, then stopping once I reached my self-imposed limit. But I was always still *hungry,* even after I'd just finished eating, and my stomach was full of low-calorie fare. Then, of course, there were always those special occasions... or in my case, homemade meals and family barbecues. I mean, how could I turn down a slice of homemade coconut pecan pie that my grandmother made from scratch?

Another factor that impedes the effectiveness of long-term caloric restriction is that our bodies eventually adapt to the limited number of calories we consume, and in turn require fewer calories to maintain our current weight. A notorious example of this biological phenomenon can be seen in a case study done on a sample of *The Biggest Loser* contestants six years after they competed on the show.[9]

Admittedly, my husband and I were huge fans of *The Biggest Loser* back in its prime. He was always Team Bob, while I was Team Jillian. Whenever I worked out, I could hear Jillian screaming in my head, "LAST CHANCE WORKOUT, PEOPLE!" I also still remember my utter excitement when Ali Vincent was the first woman to win the competition. *The Biggest Loser* made for some great reality television, but unfortunately, the contestants from the 2016 case study didn't fare so well in real life.

The study became extremely popular when the New York Times published an extensive article about it in May 2016.[10] As is typical, the contestants experienced a sharp drop in their resting metabolic rates (i.e., how many calories the body burns at rest) once they lost all that weight so quickly. What was so shocking about this particular group of individuals, though, was that their metabolisms never returned to a normal burn rate, even after the contestants regained the weight they had lost on the show. According to the article:

> *Mr. Cahill was one of the worst off. As he regained more than 100 pounds, his metabolism slowed so much that, just to maintain his current weight of 295 pounds, he now has to eat 800 calories a day less than a typical man his size. Anything more turns to fat.*

Wow. As silly as it might sound, my husband and I were a bit depressed after reading that article. I mean, if caloric restriction didn't work for *The Biggest Loser* contestants, who had the best trainers and medical experts overseeing their progress, then what did? Maybe exercise was the key to maintaining significant fat loss?

Well, a later study was also done on these participants to see whether exercise had any effect on weight loss maintenance after they left the competition.[11] Sure enough, researchers found that the contestants who continued to engage in the most physical activity were also the most successful in maintaining their weight loss. The article concluded that "large and persistent increases in [physical activity] may be required for long-term maintenance of lost weight," which amounts to *"increases of about 80 minutes"* of moderate exercise per day.[11]

Double wow! So to maintain long-term weight loss, we need to increase our physical activity by almost an hour-and-a-half per day? For someone young, single, and caring only for themselves, that might not seem like much of a stretch. In fact, I used to spend about that much time working out in my early 20s. But now as a mother who cares for three small children, works, and goes to school, I can barely find time to do laundry, let alone exercise.

To be honest, I don't even like working out or exercising like I used to. I hate going to the gym or sweating to some workout DVD in my living room. It's just not enjoyable to me. Now, I do love going on long walks, working in my garden, and taking part in many recreational outdoor activities, but I don't have the luxury of doing that every day. Who does?

Although caloric restriction and daily exercise can be effective pieces to the complex weight-loss puzzle, they alone are not enough to manage long-term weight loss. As much as we'd like to think of the human body as a well-oiled metabolic machine, it simply isn't. We are subject to thousands of biological, behavioral, and environmental cues that prompt our bodies to crave food for fuel or burn stored fuel reserves, such as body fat.

Fortunately, IF can give us a metabolic advantage by helping regulate hormones that play significant roles in hunger and metabolism.

The Hunger Hormone Games

A myriad of hormones circulating throughout our bodies affect hunger and cravings as well as fat metabolism. Although this book will not go into great detail about every single one, I think it's important to get to know some of the key players and their roles in these biological processes.

Insulin

Insulin is by far one of the major players in the role of hunger and fat metabolism. In fact, I'm inclined to call it the MVP of metabolic hormones because our bodies cannot function properly without it. This is why people afflicted with type 1 diabetes, in which the pancreas cannot produce sufficient insulin, must inject themselves regularly with a synthetic version of the hormone.

One of insulin's main jobs is to carry glucose (sugar) that is present in the blood to cells to use for energy to function. Without insulin, the body cannot burn energy from food (mostly carbohydrates) for fuel, so it will burn muscle and body fat for energy instead. In fact, no matter how much food individuals with type 1 diabetes consume, they often lose weight as a result of the body burning its own fat and muscle, instead of glucose, for fuel.

While this might sound like a dieter's dream come true, it results in dangerously high glucose levels in the blood, which can cause severe nerve and organ damage throughout the body. Hence, insulin plays a vital role in cell function and fat metabolism.

Likewise, producing too much insulin can trigger false hunger signals and keep our bodies from burning fat for fuel. And what causes too much insulin to be pumped into the body? Eating constantly throughout the day, such as with grazing and snacking, as well as eating refined or artificial carbohydrates.

Unfortunately, modern society is conducive to this overproduction of insulin. We are constantly surrounded by food and encouraged to eat as soon as we're feeling a bit peckish. For people trying to lose weight, there is a plethora of meal replacement bars and shakes that "taste great" and are chock full of protein and fiber. The problem is these fake foods are full of artificial sweeteners that the body tries to process as the real thing. One taste of that cookies 'n' cream protein bar sends insulin levels soaring in an attempt to bring down the expected spike in blood sugar, which doesn't occur due to the artificial sweeteners.

Repeating these eating patterns day after day for several years often results in symptoms of metabolic syndrome, such as weight gain, constant hunger, and insulin resistance. Some of the most easily digestible information on this topic can be found in the books *Why We Get Fat* by Gary Taubes and *The Obesity Code* by Dr. Jason Fung. If you're interested in gaining a better understanding of the role that insulin plays in our bodies, I highly recommend reading or listening to both books at your leisure.

Leptin

Leptin is another key player in the "Hunger Hormone Games," as this hormone is responsible for keeping hunger at bay. Leptin is produced primarily from fat tissue and signals the brain when the body has enough fat and energy to survive. In theory, an increase in the leptin hormone tells the body it's full, and a decrease in leptin tells the body to eat.

When researchers discovered in the early 1950s that leptin-deficient mice became morbidly obese, they hoped that cloning this hormone could serve as a cure for obesity. However, scientists soon discovered that obese people actually produce *higher* levels of leptin than their non-obese counterparts do, and eventually they develop leptin resistance. Much like what happens when individuals are insulin resistant, the body produces more and more leptin to signal that it is full, but instead causes "exaggerated brain responses in the motivation-reward pathways, which in turn increases the risk of overconsumption and loss of eating control."[12]

Not surprisingly, leptin levels drop during periods of fasting. This makes sense since the body eventually requires food for energy, and dwindling levels of leptin signal hunger to the brain. This may sound like bad news for someone who wants to try fasting, since the last thing we want is to feel hungry during a fast. What's surprising is that fasting also helps the body become more sensitive to leptin, which means less leptin hormone is needed to help us feel sated.[13]

Research showed that microbes in the gut may be responsible for mediating the release of leptin into the body. Obese people produce less of this microbe, which makes them resistant to leptin, causing them to produce more and more leptin to try and keep the body satiated. Fasting allows the gut to recoup and regenerate various microbes and peptides that aid in the metabolic process and regulate hunger.[14]

Ghrelin

Ghrelin is the "grumpy gremlin" of metabolic hormones. This hormone is responsible for telling the brain "Feed me!" So, if you've ever felt "hangry," you can be sure that ghrelin was at play. Ghrelin levels rise sharply at anticipated meal and snack times, then slowly decline after the meal is eaten. However, studies found that other factors, such as lack of sleep, stress, and even tasty snacks, can increase ghrelin and hunger signals.[15–17]

As if that didn't make weight-loss difficult enough, studies also found that reducing caloric intake and losing weight both result in increased levels of ghrelin[18, 19], which in turn increases hunger signals and makes food taste even more delicious.[20] This is not a good combination of factors for anyone trying to lose weight by cutting calories.

However, some studies showed that various forms of IF often decrease hunger signals and do not impact ghrelin levels negatively.[14, 21] Ghrelin levels, in fact, steadily decrease over the course of a 24-hour fast, just after the first few spikes associated with scheduled meal times.[22] And fasting for 72 hours has been shown to completely eliminate "meal-related ghrelin secretion," in essence resetting the body's hunger cues.[21]

Of course, several other hormones, such as cortisol, estrogen, and thyroxine, affect hunger and satiety, but insulin, leptin, and ghrelin are three key players that directly affect our hunger signals. IF can help regulate these hunger hormones so we can lose weight naturally without feeling hungry all the time.

It's vitally important, however, that we ease into the process and allow our bodies and minds to adjust to this new way of eating. The next chapter will explain exactly how to do that.

MIND OVER BODY

Although the What IF Diet Plan will eventually free you from having to worry about food or exercise, having a solid plan is crucial for getting started. Therefore, you will have to think about food and do some minor planning for at least the first few weeks of the plan. I promise it will be much simpler than most of the popular diets you may have tried in the past.

Phase 1: Push It Back, Then Bring It In

First off, if you have been eating every three to four hours throughout your life like most people, you are probably thinking that there's *no way* you can go eight or more hours without eating and not feel ravenous. The truth is, you're probably right. Now, I don't say this to discourage you, but to prepare you for the transition phase of the What IF Diet Plan.

If you are used to eating every few hours, your body is also used to utilizing food and calories for fuel. It will take some time to deplete your glycogen stores so your body can become adept at using its own fat for fuel, a concept often referred to as being *fat adapted*.

Becoming fat adapted takes some time, but is totally worth it for anyone trying to lose weight, gain energy, and take control of their eating.

So, how do you get started with fasting when you're not fat adapted?

Well, it turns out we're already fasting every day, whether we realize it or not. When we sleep for several hours at night, we are truly fasting. Conventional advice tells us that going to sleep with a full stomach is not healthy because our bodies cannot digest food during this time or burn calories efficiently, which means excess calories will be transformed to excess fat. However, this is also the peak time that human growth hormone is released in the body, which is necessary for cell growth and repair. In fact, sleep is imperative for fat and calorie burning, as well as for allowing the body to heal itself naturally.

Conventional wisdom also tells us that breakfast is the most important meal of the day. While there is some truth to this, it does not mean that breakfast must be eaten immediately upon waking. Popular diets advise us to eat breakfast within an hour after waking to *jumpstart the metabolism* and *keep our metabolism burning throughout the day*. Again, while breakfast does provide a slight upsurge in calorie burn, it's not a significant factor in overall calorie burn for the day. Also, breakfast provides this jumpstart to the metabolism whether you eat breakfast at eight in the morning or eight in the evening. Eating breakfast simply means you are eating your first meal of the day and "breaking" your "fast."

Therefore, rather than skipping breakfast altogether, I suggest simply pushing it back to a later time. Choose a time that is *challenging,* yet *realistic* given your current hunger cues, lifestyle, and schedule. For example, if you're attending a conference that offers breakfast at eight in the morning and a coffee break with snacks at ten, try sleeping in or taking a morning walk during breakfast, attending your conference as usual, then making the coffee break your first meal of the day. Luckily, fasting and pushing back regularly scheduled meals is much easier when you are busy.

Personally, I used to eat breakfast at 7:15 with my kids, then grab a snack from the vending machine or nearby Starbucks around 10 a.m. every day. It was usually something "healthy," such as a bag of mixed nuts, low-fat yogurt, or a low-calorie breakfast sandwich, which I felt kept my metabolism burning until lunchtime. So to fit the What IF Diet Plan in my personal schedule, I decided I would forgo my usual breakfast, and simply eat my real breakfast at 10 when my coworkers and I partook in our regular morning snack. However, I still drank my usual coffee with heavy cream and sugar-free vanilla sweetener throughout the morning.

The first few days of pushing back breakfast can be a struggle. Even if you're not a fan of breakfast, your stomach is probably used to having something sitting in there to keep it quiet. At times, your stomach may even growl and throw tantrums like a fussy toddler! This is also about the time that those unfounded thoughts will come creeping into your mind. Your mind will tell you that you are putting undue stress on your body, ruining your metabolism, or causing a sugar crash! When your mind and body are both prodding you in this manner, it is tempting to give in and eat the first food you find to soothe your inner toddler.

I learned to disrupt my thoughts during these times and ask myself:

What IF my body is not starving?

What IF my body is just adjusting to something new?

What IF pushing back breakfast is allowing my body some necessary recovery time?

What IF I could learn to stop associating food with pleasure and punishment?

I realized that after repeating these mental mantras to myself several times, and sometimes distracting myself by briefly walking around or chatting with a coworker, the hunger pangs would become subdued. In fact, they often lasted no more than 90 seconds... although it might feel like an eternity when you're hungry.

So, your first step to starting the What IF Diet Plan is to push your breakfast back, even if it's only by an hour or two. You can still drink coffee, preferably black, as well as water and unsweetened tea. If you must have creamer with your coffee or tea, I recommend just a splash of real heavy cream and cinnamon, rather than a sugar-free flavored creamer, if possible. We will touch on the reasons for these recommendations in a later chapter, *Fine-Tune Your Fasting*.

And when those sabotaging thoughts enter your mind, I encourage you to come up with your own "What IF?" questions to ask yourself. This exercise may feel silly, but the questions you choose to ask yourself about this plan are critical to your success. Asking good "What IF?" questions helps you focus on your goal and steer clear of discouraging mental chatter. If you're unable to come up with your own questions now, then feel free to use the ones I asked myself:

What IF

_____

_____ ?

What IF

_____

_____ ?

What IF

_____

_____ ?

What IF

_____

_____ ?

What IF

_____

_____?

Now, Bring It In

Now that you've decided on a set time to eat breakfast, let's look at our last meal of the day, which is most likely *not* dinner. If you're anything like me, you might want a little something sweet, salty, or alcoholic after eating a good dinner—even if you're "not hungry." Rather than denying yourself that nighttime snack, we're going to consider this our last meal of the day. Personally, I love having a glass of wine with fruit, popcorn, a bowl of cereal, or a comforting ham and cheese sandwich. As you can imagine, these kinds of nighttime snacks can really add to the waistline if you're eating throughout the entire day.

Since we have set a new time to eat our breakfast, however, we can now calculate when our last meal should be. Ideally, you want to plan to stop eating within 12 hours of your first meal. Therefore, if you ate your breakfast at nine in the morning, you should plan to stop eating no later than nine that night. This time frame of eating is referred to as your *eating window*. Any time outside this window when you are not eating is referred to as your *fasting window*.

I know what you might be thinking if you have already read about or tried IF in the past: *Aren't you supposed to eat within an eight-*

hour eating window? Well, yes... in a perfect world, that's what a beginning intermittent faster should aim for. Fast for 16 hours and eat all snacks and meals within eight hours. On the What IF Diet Plan, though, I highly recommend that you aim to fast for 12 hours and allow yourself 12 hours to eat all meals and snacks.

I make this recommendation because it's hard for someone who is dependent on continual energy from food to stick to an eight-hour eating window. Most likely, you will go to bed hungry and wake up *starving*, then feel frustrated and betrayed by your own body, which often leads to emotional eating. So let's skip all the drama and aim for simple and doable 12-hour fasting/eating windows.

If you stop eating prior to the end of your eating window, then you can open your eating window earlier the next day if needed. Likewise, if you need to open your eating window earlier for professional or personal reasons (e.g., an early morning work meeting or breakfast with the in-laws), then aim to stop eating within 12 hours of doing so. Not eating after 8 or 9 p.m. is much more achievable than not eating after 4 or 5 p.m. So again, strive for 12-hour fasting and eating windows each day for the next three weeks.

Trust the Plan, Not the Scale

The first phase of the What IF Diet Plan is *not* about losing weight fast, gaining energy, lowering blood sugar, or achieving mental clarity throughout the day—although those side effects often occur during this time. Instead, the plan is about creating an effective, healthy, and worry-free way of eating that you can fit into your lifestyle. If you're used to eating several times throughout the day and dive headfirst into a 16-hour fast, you are setting yourself up for failure.

People who try fasting for extended periods without prior practice often experience something called *compensatory eating*. It happens when the following items occur simultaneously:

1. Your body believes that you have encountered a famine, and you need to eat more to store excess calories as energy that can be used later (i.e., glycogen and body fat).

2. Your mind believes that since you've been "good" all day, you "deserve" to eat more to compensate for the calories that you missed out on throughout the day.

While these mind-body processes are meant to help us survive and thrive, they are both misguided and not fruitful in our modern-day lifestyles. Plus, while compensatory eating is temporary and usually subsides after a few weeks (or months) of consistent IF, it can lead to feeling sluggish and bloated at the end of your eating window, and to weight gain. Although I argue that some weight gain is not bad, it can be discouraging and make you feel worse than before.

To circumvent this cycle of white-knuckle fasting and compensatory eating, the first phase of the What IF Diet Plan requires you to focus on maintaining 12-hour fasting and eating windows for three weeks... and that's it! At this point in the plan, we are training our minds and bodies to ignore some of their usual hunger cues, and re-learn what real hunger and energy feel like. Are you really *hungry* for a sausage-egg-and-cheese-biscuit sandwich and Frappuccino at 7:30 in the morning? Does eating that early really provide you with the energy you need to get through the day? Is it really going to kill you to push your breakfast back by a couple of hours?

For the first week or two, your mind and body will be screaming "YES! Get in my belly!" However, I guarantee that by week three, you will catch yourself wondering why you ever bothered eating so early in the first place. You may also notice other small mental and biological shifts, such as physically feeling your stomach growl, but realizing that you're not that hungry. Or catching yourself working through your newly scheduled breakfast time because you're so mentally focused on something other than food. If you find this happening during the first phase, you can certainly push back your eating window further, by an hour or so, if you wish.

During the first phase of the What IF Diet Plan, I also recommend that you *do not* weigh yourself. The plan involves changing the way you think about food, nutrition, exercise, and *especially* body weight. Although body weight can be an indicator of health, it is only one small piece of an extremely complex puzzle we know as the human body. Regrettably, society has taught us to view weight as a concrete measure of our success. Losing 10 pounds is considered a win, whereas gaining 10 pounds is considered a colossal failure—especially for women.

Personally, I weighed myself every day for the first couple of weeks of my What IF Diet Plan. I was ecstatic when I first lost three pounds in two days! Then pissed off when I gained five pounds over the next couple of days after that. Throughout the first couple of weeks, I was so frustrated with the numbers on my scale that I decided to quit and chalk IF up to another fad, once again.

I was thankful that small voice of reason piped up at just the right time:

What IF...? What IF the number on the scale is not an accurate indicator of my success?

What IF the other benefits of intermittent fasting are still worth striving for?

*What IF I just stopped weighing myself altogether? *Gasp!**

With these new "What IF?" questions, I was also forced to remind myself of the three conditions I had previously agreed would factor into whether I stuck to the What IF Diet Plan:

1. It could not interfere with my family, work, or social life.

2. It had to be convenient and cost effective.

3. I would not take part in any form of exercise or physical activity that I did not enjoy.

Nowhere in these conditions did I say, "I must not gain weight." Plus, I'd read countless research articles and watched numerous videos and documentaries about the benefits of fasting. Why should gaining a few pounds detract from that? Besides, I was trying this new way of living to improve my overall health, not to look like a supermodel.

At that point I decided to *trust the plan, not the scale*. As tempted as I was to use the scale as a visual measure of my success on the What IF Diet Plan, I realized it was only sabotaging my progress. Therefore, I made a pact to forgo the scale for at least one month and focus on maintaining my eating and fasting windows instead. If I met my fasting/ eating window goals, I would consider myself successful for that day.

Now, what "What IF?" questions can you ask yourself to determine your measure of success that does not depend on a number on the scale?:

What IF

_____

_____ ?

What IF

_____

_____ ?

What IF

_____

_____ ?

What IF

_____

_____ ?

What IF

_____

_____ ?

Phase 2: **Shrink Your Eating Window**

Now that you've stuck to 12-hour fasting and eating windows for at least three weeks, it should be fairly easy to be faithful to them. Sure, you might be tempted by the occasional office doughnut run or weekend splurge, but overall you should feel good. If you're still feeling extremely hungry before it's time to open your eating window, you can continue practicing IF with 12-hour windows for another few weeks, until this pattern feels effortless.

If you are still feeling extreme hunger during a 12-hour fasting window after six weeks of practice, there may be other factors upsetting your hunger and satiety signals. To look further into these factors, see the chapter titled *Fine-Tuning Your Fasting*.

If you're able to stick to 12-hour fasting and eating windows with little effort, then it's time for Phase 2 of the What IF Diet Plan: Shrink Your Eating Window, which is as simple as it sounds. Aim to shrink your eating window by two to three hours a day over the next three weeks.

So, if you are used to eating within a 12-hour eating window, you'll want to reduce it to 9-10 hours long. You can achieve a smaller eating window by pushing your breakfast back by another hour or two, or by "closing" your eating window earlier than usual. Or you can try a combination of the two—whatever works best for your way of living!

During this phase of the What IF Diet Plan, I struggled to shrink my window by forgoing my nightly snack. I told myself that it was just empty calories, and that it wasn't healthy for me to eat so close to bedtime. Since I had mastered my 12-hour windows, it was rare that I ever ate past 9 p.m., so I figured that closing my window by seven would be a piece of cake. If I really wanted my evening snack, I could just eat it earlier.

I continued to open my window at 10 a.m. for the next week, despite not feeling hungry, and told myself that I would stop eating by 7 p.m. As usual, the first couple of days went without a hitch. I really missed my normal bedtime snack, but knew I was doing my body well by eating it earlier or skipping it altogether.

Unfortunately, by day three, I was miserable and grumpy. All I wanted was to sip a glass of wine or hot tea with honey and munch on something after taking a hot shower and settling into bed after a long day. Was that so wrong? I scolded myself, saying, "You can't be physically hungry at 9 p.m. if you ate dinner two hours ago. Suck it up buttercup!"

My school and personal schedule also made it difficult to stop eating by seven. I had a night class from 6 to 8:30 every Wednesday, which meant I either had to scarf down dinner before class or skip it altogether. Obviously, I was not happy with either of these options. Most nights, I didn't get home with the kids until after seven, which made it impossible to eat dinner early, unless I ate in the car.

After a week of trying to adjust to my newly mandated eating window, I figured that it was time to reevaluate my strategy. I indeed wanted to shrink my eating window and expand my fasting window incrementally, but maybe I was going about it the wrong way. I soon realized that I was again not abiding by my own agreements for following my What IF Diet Plan:

1. It could not interfere with my family, work, or social life.

2. It had to be convenient and cost effective.

3. I would not take part in any form of exercise or physical activity that I did not enjoy.

By denying myself of my beloved bedtime snack, I was causing unnecessary stress on myself and my family, which went against agreement number 1. Trying to cram dinner in before seven was *not* convenient for my schedule. Plus, picking something up on the go, rather than simply cooking and enjoying a late dinner, was not cost-effective. So why was I so intent on closing my window early if it clearly wasn't working for me? I asked myself more "What IF?" questions:

What IF eating after 7 p.m. was not bad for me?

What IF eating right before bed was not the cardinal dietary sin I thought it was?

What IF our bodies can burn and utilize late-night food just as effectively as food eaten earlier in the day?

After asking myself these questions and reevaluating my beliefs around optimal eating times, I decided to push my eating window back by a couple of hours instead, from noon to 10 p.m. I ate breakfast and lunch at work, then a late dinner at home, and allowed myself to have a snack before bed. This eating window worked much better for my crazy schedule. I didn't feel rushed to eat meals at inconvenient times, and was able to relax and spend quality time with my husband before bed.

Eventually, my eating window naturally shrank on its own. Since work kept me busy, I often noticed that I wasn't hungry at my usual eating time. Where I was normally opening my eating window at noon, I often continued working through that time, not realizing that it was "lunchtime" already. Sometimes I would still eat because I feared that I would not have time to eat later, but eventually I listened to my hunger cues and took heed.

Every couple of weeks, I noticed myself getting hungry later and later in the day. After a few months, I started getting hungry and opening my window around 3 p.m. Although this shift seemingly occurred without effort, it would not have happened had I not challenged my beliefs about eating at night. In fact, I was ready to quit IF... again!

If you find yourself feeling defeated or stressed out by long-held food or body beliefs, it may be time to come up with some good "What IF?" questions to ask yourself as well:

What IF

_____

_____ ?

What IF

_____

_____ ?

What IF

_____

_____ ?

What IF

_____

_____ ?

"So When Do You Eat?"

If your job is like mine, you most likely have a scheduled lunch hour. In our office, staff members go to lunch at noon. Although our boss allows some flexibility, requesting a lunch hour at 3 p.m. didn't seem plausible or enjoyable to me. So, what in the world was I supposed to do at noon if I wasn't eating?

Most days I would continue working or catch up on homework, which was nice since the office was empty and quiet. I soon realized, though, that my brain needed a break from working on a computer all day. To give myself a mental break, I tried doing other activities, such as reading a book, yoga, meditating, swimming, and even taking a cat nap. Although I normally find these activities enjoyable, it wasn't the same when trying to cram them into one hour. Maybe working through lunch wasn't so bad after all.

One day, I decided to stretch my legs and take a 10-minute walk around campus to clear my mind. The South Texas heat can be brutal in the spring and summer months, so I didn't want to be outside long. As I walked, though, I could feel the stress and tension melt away from my mind and body. I felt surprisingly refreshed and ready to the take on the rest of the day when I returned to the office.

Before I knew it, I was walking every day during my scheduled lunch hour. The 10-minute walk eventually increased to the entire hour, which added up to about two miles. I am fortunate to work on a beautiful college campus that's perfect for walking, and I always wore a giant sunhat and sunscreen to protect my skin. Although these walks were good for my physical health, I found them just as good for my mental health as well.

Eventually, colleagues around campus would see me walking and began asking about my "workout" routine. I found it awkward explaining that walking was more for my mental health than physical health because I still viewed physical activity and exercise as a tool for burning calories. Inevitably, the next question would be, "So when do you eat?" Another awkward question.

Although IF is now widely accepted, it was still somewhat taboo back in 2018. I think this is especially true in certain cultures. In the Hispanic culture, food is used to nourish our loved ones, celebrate milestones, mourn deaths, cure ailments, show love, and everything in between. When I was growing up, Abuelita (Grandma) constantly asked if we were hungry, and always had pastries and sweet bread available to nibble on. Refusing food was cause for alarm and meant that you were feeling ill or on some crazy crash diet. It is also extremely rude and disrespectful to turn away food from your abuela, so I wouldn't dare!

Although South Texas culture is changing, many old-school beliefs about food and eating remain. So, when people asked me, "When do you eat your lunch?" I'd explain that I was trying something called intermittent fasting in which I don't eat consistently throughout the day. I'd tell them I was listening to my body's natural hunger cues and noticed that I wasn't hungry at noon anymore, so I ate my "lunch" around three when I *was* hungry.

The most common comment people would make was, "Oh, I could never do that! I would be *starving* by lunchtime!" I'd then talk about how I started by simply pushing my breakfast back one hour at a time and noticed that my hunger naturally shifted. I'd also mention all the benefits I'd experienced, such as more energy, mental clarity, steady weight loss, clearer skin, and how convenient it was not to have to think about food all the time. At that point in the conversation, I'd often get a "Huh... that sounds pretty good. I might try that someday." True to their word, many of the people I've spoken to about IF have tried it and effortlessly adapted it to their own personal lifestyle.

Phase 3: **Watch Yourself**

Phase 3 of the What IF Diet Plan actually begins at Phase 1, but most people find it difficult to identify the destructive thoughts and beliefs they have around food, weight, and health. I know I did. People want step-by-step instructions on *how* to change and want to see evidence of change before they'll believe it's possible. Once they see proof that it "works," then they will give themselves the credit they deserved all along.

Throughout my What IF Diet Plan journey, I realized that the thoughts and beliefs I had about myself were just as important (if not more so) than sticking to my eating window or eating healthy foods. There were many times I believed this lifestyle was too good to be true, or that I would end up gaining all my weight back, or that I couldn't keep up IF forever. While these thoughts seem harmless, and somewhat reasonable, they often resulted in unnecessary worry and self-sabotage.

For example, on Sunday mornings, my husband and I enjoy cooking a large brunch for the family, usually consisting of French toast, berries, eggs, bacon, sausage, hash browns, etc. For the first few weeks of fasting, I gladly ate brunch with the family since it fit in perfectly with my 12-hour eating window. However, eating brunch became less enjoyable as my hunger naturally delayed later and later. After a few months, eating brunch made me feel sick and lethargic for the rest of the day.

The thought of sitting on the sidelines awkwardly sipping black coffee while my family sat at the kitchen table eating and talking sounded miserable. As a mom, I felt I needed to set a good example for my boys by joining them at the table and eating with the family. I started thinking, *I knew this was too good to be true*, and *I can't allow IF to interfere with family time*, and *It's not good for my boys to see me only drinking coffee all day*. While these thoughts might seem silly, they were insidious and kept me from trusting my body's natural signals.

Once again, I found myself questioning my beliefs, but this time it wasn't just about food and health. I was now questioning beliefs that could impact my family, which I found problematic. Finally, I decided to ask myself better "What IF?" questions about my dilemma rather than drowning in guilt-inducing mental chatter:

What IF I could still join the family for brunch without eating?

What IF following my natural hunger cues was setting a healthy example for my kids?

What IF my kids cared more about having me at the table than whether I ate?

What IF not eating Sunday brunch with the family doesn't make me a "bad" mom?

At this point in my What IF Diet Plan journey, you would think the answers to these questions were obvious, although I find that it's more difficult to notice sneaky thoughts and question deceptive beliefs when it's yourself doing the thinking. These types of examples reminded me of a quote from Eckhart Tolle's book *The Power of Now*:

> *To disidentify from thinking is to be the silent watcher of your thoughts and behavior, especially the repetitive patterns of your mind and the roles played by the ego.*

Even though I'd read this book at least three times over the years, I finally realized what it meant to put Tolle's words into action. I also realized how scary and powerful it can be to be the "watcher of your thoughts" and notice the "repetitive patterns" and "roles" we play out. After having children, my focus was always on family.

I'd gotten better about participating in self-care activities, such as meditating, walking, and taking long baths, but I still had a tough time agreeing to anything that might put my needs before my family's.

This is when I realized that the most important phase of the What IF Diet Plan is to *watch yourself*. On days when I find myself thinking unhelpful, worrisome, or anxious thoughts, I do my best to take a break and watch myself. If I'm really struggling or having trouble identifying my troublesome thoughts, I write them down. The surprising thing is that as I'm writing down my thoughts, my brain often comes up with solutions or helpful "What IF?" questions to challenge myself with.

On those days that I "don't have time" to write down thoughts (or if I'm being completely honest, just don't feel like it!) I stop, take a deep breath, and tell myself, "Girl, you better watch yourself!" Immediately, I'm reminded of how important our mindsets and beliefs are to living our best lives. Likewise, when I'm questioning my ability to do something, I'll come up with at least three helpful "What IF?" questions instead of dwelling on my stinkin' thinkin'.

PRACTICE MAKES ~~PERFECT~~ POSSIBLE

We've all heard the phrase "practice makes perfect." Personally, I've never been a fan of this term because although I believe that practice is crucial for learning a new skill or habit, perfection is rarely attainable. Striving for perfection often results in self-sabotage, insecurity, and, ultimately, failure when we do not achieve it.

For years I strived for perfection when trying out a new diet plan or setting new goals for myself. As soon as things did not go the way they were supposed to, I'd label myself a "failure" doomed to be overweight for the rest of my life. I followed similar self-defeating patterns in other areas of my life as well.

If I could not present an idea to my boss perfectly, then I wouldn't present it at all. Then I'd feel discouraged when I was passed up for a promotion. If I couldn't write a perfect research paper, then I wouldn't bother turning it in and got an F instead. If I couldn't stick to a 16-hour fasting window, then I considered myself weak-willed and wrote IF off as another fad diet.

As I followed my What IF Diet Plan, though, I realized that there is no perfect way to fast or eat that would lead me to dietary nirvana. On some days I'm ravenous by noon, and on other days I'm not hungry until 7 p.m. On some days I eat a salad and protein for dinner, and on other days I eat a sandwich with chips and a doughnut (maybe three)... and that's OK. I've learned that beating myself up for not being "perfect" makes me feel horrible and results in missing opportunities for growth and improvement. Therefore, I continue to practice IF and watch my thoughts, but no longer strive for "perfection."

So let's forget the phrase "practice makes perfect" because it's simply not true. Instead, focus on *practice makes possible* because the more you practice IF and challenging your own limiting beliefs, the more you will realize what's possible for your life. Watch yourself and be conscious of how you think about your life. When you catch yourself thinking discouraging or self-defeating thoughts, stop and come up with some helpful "What IF?" questions to challenge those thoughts with.

Asking good "What IF?" questions allows your mind to focus on what's possible, rather than the obstacles that lie in your way. In fact, you may find that those obstacles don't even exist! A good example of this is when I questioned myself about eating brunch with the family. I believed that a good mother should join her family in eating brunch, and that not eating was setting a bad example for my children.

In this scenario, the impediments that I had about parenting and setting a good example for my kids were really non-existent. By asking myself useful "What IF?" questions about my perceptions, I was able to challenge my ingrained beliefs and discover solutions to self-imposed problems. I encourage and challenge you to do the same.

What IF

_____

_____ ?

What IF

_____

_____ ?

What IF

_____

_____ ?

What IF

_____

_____ ?

What IF

_____

_____ ?

WEIGHT LOSS IS A SIDE EFFECT

A major reason that I was driven to continue following my What IF Diet Plan was because I wanted to reap all benefits that IF has to offer. After several months of practicing IF, I realized that weight loss was simply another positive side effect of IF and gaining overall good health. Indeed, there is a multitude of research articles and anecdotal evidence on how IF makes people feel more energized, subdues cravings, increases mental clarity, improves the immune system, and so much more.

Superhuman Energy

When I started IF, I was afraid of feeling weak and sluggish due to not eating consistently throughout the day. For the first few weeks of pushing my breakfast back, this indeed felt like the case. However, after several weeks of stretching the time before having breakfast and fasting for 12 hours a day, I realized that I actually felt more energized than usual. It reminded me of my younger days when I flitted around like a hummingbird on steroids... and it felt great! I'd always attributed this steady stream of energy to all the coffee I drank during that time, but maybe there was more to it.

As I researched more about the benefits of IF, I quickly realized that feeling more energized was indeed a welcome side effect of fasting. When we eat continuously throughout the day, our bodies are accustomed to converting that food into energy. Therefore, we often feel irritable or like we have low blood sugar if we go longer than usual without eating. This is also why it's difficult for people to start IF with a 16-hour fasting window right off the bat. Fortunately, as we continue to practice fasting, our bodies learn to become less reliant on food for energy and begin using our own fat for fuel. This process is often referred to as being fat adapted, which was briefly discussed in the Mind Over Body chapter.

Once my body became fat adapted, I felt as if I could do or accomplish anything! I directed all my newfound energy toward work, family, school, and home improvement projects. During the week I'd work a full day, take the kids to football practice, and still have enough energy to cook dinner and help with homework afterward. On the weekends I began doing yard work and home improvement projects, which I'd previously considered my husband's responsibility. Housework and homework also became easier for me to keep up with and manage.

Some days I'd mentally marvel at the strength and energy I exerted throughout the day. I felt as if I had superhuman energy because it was not produced by an energy drink, pill, or power bar. My body produced it entirely on its own. And best of all, this energy was being supplied by excess unwanted body fat!

Reduced Hunger and Mental Chatter About Food

My favorite side effect of practicing IF was that I stopped feeling distracted by hunger and food all day. Have you ever finished eating a full meal only to feel "hungry" less than an hour later? Logically, you know that you can't be hungry so soon after eating, but that doesn't change that you still feel hungry.

Before practicing IF, I was constantly hungry throughout the day. On the rare occasions that I wasn't hungry, I was always thinking about what I would eat for my next meal or snack. While following previous diets or just counting calories, I would think about what combinations of foods I could eat to stay within my dietary restrictions. My head was flooded with questions and calculations about what foods, supplements, or beverages I could consume to squelch my never-ending hunger but still help me "not gain weight."

I'd have a stash of pre-cooked meatballs, chicken, roasted veggies, boiled eggs, bacon, etc. on hand when I was eating low carb so I wouldn't be tempted to eat anything off my plan. If I was calorie counting, I would play with different combinations of foods in my calorie counting app to see what I could eat and still stay within 1,500 calories per day. If my latest diet plan allowed a cheat day, I would daydream about all the junk I would get to eat on that day if I was "good" during the week.

As mentioned in the *Mind Over Body* chapter, my hunger cues slowly shifted to later in the day after several weeks of consistently practicing IF. It didn't happen overnight, but once it did, I was in awe! It had been years since I could remember not feeling hungry or distracted by thoughts of food. Again, it reminded me of the days when I was practicing IF and not realizing it. I'd be so focused on school or work that I'd continue working into my eating window several times throughout the week.

With that, I would like to share a quick anecdote, and if you've ever felt out of control with your hunger, I think you will relate. You see, I work on a large college campus, and my office building is across the street from a dining hall where students can pick up various fast-food items. One of the favorite dining options is a restaurant called Chick-fil-A, which serves amazing southern-style chicken sandwiches and nuggets—and waffle fries. If you're lucky enough to live near a Chick-fil-A restaurant, then you know what I'm talking about!

As you may remember, a few months into practicing my What IF Diet Plan, I started taking walks during my lunch hour, then eating lunch in my office afterward once my eating window opened. One afternoon, I decided to switch up my walking route and ended up passing the dining hall that I normally avoided due to heavy foot traffic. Before I knew it, the smell of waffle fries and fried chicken wafted into my nostrils. I immediately regretted this decision and braced myself for some intense stomach rumblings. To my surprise, though, my stomach didn't rumble.

I walked right by the dining hall, smelled the delicious food, but didn't feel the crazy hunger cues I normally did. My stomach didn't growl. My mouth didn't water. Surely this had to be a fluke. As ridiculous as it sounds, I decided to test this new wondrous sensation of non-hunger further by turning around and passing the dining hall again. The same thing happened.

I'm sure I looked like a crazy person. I literally stood in front of the dining hall for a good 30 seconds just inhaling all the wonderful fried-food smells and waiting for hunger to pounce from the shadows like El Cucuy! But it didn't. I was able to smell and appreciate the food without feeling like I had to have it.

I was so excited about this new milestone in my IF endeavor that I called my husband just to tell him what had happened. He sounded confused but gave me a half-hearted congratulations for whatever it was that I was so excited about. Once I got back to my building, I burst into my coworker's office and told her about my exhilarating discovery. She politely congratulated me as well.

As silly as this story may sound, I consider it a personal milestone for my physical and mental health. For so many years I felt as if I were a prisoner to food and hunger. I'd felt like my body was punishing me for years of yo-yo dieting and skipping meals in my younger days, when it was actually just as confused as I was. Practicing IF allowed my body's hunger hormones to recalibrate, essentially resetting my hunger cues as well. It was at this point in my What IF Diet journey that I knew IF was right for me.

Improved Cognitive Function

Improved cognitive function is often another side effect of practicing IF. When I experienced what felt like enhanced mental clarity after fasting several hours, I wasn't sure if it was attributable to IF. I'd also adopted other healthy habits, such as meditating, drinking black coffee, walking, and journaling, so I knew it may well have been a culmination of these new habits combined. However, there is a great deal of research that supports the notion that fasting can improve cognitive function.

A comprehensive article in the Journal of Neuroscience provides an in-depth report of many ways that fasting impacts cognitive function. For example, when the body is deprived of food for long periods, most organs decrease in size—but not the brain.[23] IF is also associated with improved synaptic plasticity and increased production of neurons.[23, 24] One study even found that IF reduced impulsivity and increased accuracy in a group of professional cyclists during the weeks of Ramadan fasting.[25] It's thought that these processes may occur because high-level cognitive function was once necessary for survival when food was scarce. [23, 24]

Personally, I believe one reason I experienced improved cognitive function and overall well-being with IF is because I stopped wasting my mental energy on thinking about food. I still consider myself a foodie and look forward to my meals, but I'm not obsessing over when, how much, or what I should eat. I try to plan healthy meals for my family, but if we get takeout a couple of nights a week, I no longer consider it a failure on my part. I also don't worry about counting carbs, calories, points, etc. I eat what my family eats and make modifications as I see fit.

Nowadays I use my improved cognitive function to focus on more significant aspects of my life, such as family time, school, and work. I enjoy planning family vacations, researching for my homework assignments and term papers, and thinking of new initiatives for my workplace. Of course, I've also focused my energy on writing this book, which I feel is vital in sharing the wonderful effects of IF.

Autophagy

Autophagy is by far one of the greatest benefits of IF! It is essentially the body's natural process of purging or repairing damaged cells and regenerating healthy ones. Autophagy has been associated with many desirable cosmetic benefits, such as weight loss, hair regrowth, tightening loose skin, and fading stretchmarks and age spots. It is also connected with significant health matters, including reducing inflammation, eliminating toxins, shrinking fibroids, and inhibiting cancer growth.

Autophagy is a natural protective measure of the body induced by stress to help our cells adapt to new demanding environments. In the "caveman days," such stress may have been in the form of running from predators or going several days without food. However, a plentitude of research shows that autophagy can also be induced by exercise and IF.

In my view, autophagy is like the shiny golden egg of health and wellness. We all want it, but don't want to work too hard to get it. However, by practicing IF, your body essentially becomes its own golden goose, able to lay golden eggs daily without much effort!

As excited as I get about the side effects of autophagy in IF, I'm not providing a great deal of information about it here because there are experts who can explain its benefits more eloquently than I can. If you're interested in learning more about autophagy, I highly recommend that you read *The Obesity Code* by Dr. Jason Fung or *The Longevity Diet* by Dr. Valter Longo. Dr. Longo also provides a generous list of his fascinating research articles on autophagy and disease on his website.

Weight Loss

Finally, the side effect everyone's been waiting for: weight loss! Weight loss is probably the most common reason people try IF. It, or the lack of it, may also be the most common reason they give up on IF. In my own experience, weight loss was not an immediate result of practicing IF—at least not in my mind.

As mentioned in *Trust the Plan, Not the Scale*, I weighed myself every day the first two weeks of starting IF, and was incredibly frustrated when I didn't lose any weight. I'd compare myself to how I was in my younger days when weight seemed to fall off when I was IF-ing in error. I couldn't understand why it wasn't happening now.

Upon further reflection though, I realized that weight loss was never my primary goal during those times that I implemented IF in high school or in my early 20s. I executed IF more out of convenience because I didn't feel like getting up early to make breakfast, and because I felt like I had superhuman energy throughout the day, and because I wasn't hungry and didn't think about food until dinner. Sure I lost weight, but the weight loss was simply a side effect of practicing IF for its other benefits.

I was intrigued when I heard about IF in 2010 via *Eat Stop Eat* and the "5:2 Diet" because it seemed like a great way to lose the last 15 pounds of baby weight. Plus, I used to skip breakfast and lunch years before, so I figured it wouldn't be so hard. Wrong! After years of eating small meals throughout the day, jumping headfirst into a 16-hour fast was a total nightmare! I felt hungry and shaky the entire day, then binged on something—anything—at dinnertime. There was no way I could keep it up or lose weight eating that way. After two days of trying to fast for 16 hours, I gave up and moved on to the next diet scheme.

This time my start to IF was similar, in that I wanted to lose weight, but had a major difference from my unsuccessful attempt in 2010. This time I continued practicing it for all the other benefits it offered. I was also adamant about sticking to the agreements I made with myself about whether I would stick with my What IF Diet Plan:

1. It could not interfere with my family, work, or social life.

2. It had to be convenient and cost effective.

3. I would not take part in any form of exercise or physical activity that I did not enjoy.

Once I stopped focusing on weight loss and started concentrating on creating a realistic diet plan that worked for me and my family, guess what happened? The weight just fell off! Or at least that's what it felt like. In reality, I lost about 30 pounds after four months of practicing IF and asking myself helpful "What IF?" questions.

As I practiced shrinking my eating window and watching myself for pesky unfounded beliefs, I began to reap all the rewards that IF offers. I had more strength, energy, and improved mental clarity, spent less time planning meals, and found it extremely convenient and cost-effective. After carrying out The What IF? Diet Plan since 2018, I have realized that weight loss was always just a side effect.

FINE-TUNE YOUR FASTING

At this point in your What IF Diet Plan journey, you should have the basic strategies of IF down. I hope you have already experienced some great results, such as your clothes fitting looser, reduced hunger pangs throughout the day, more energy, and clearer skin.

If you haven't experienced the great benefits of fasting, or your progress has dwindled over time, it may be time to fine-tune your fasts. People often sabotage their fasting unintentionally by consuming certain items during their fasting window or overindulging once it's time to open their eating window. Fortunately, to make the What IF Diet Plan more successful and effortless we can use a couple of simple tricks that I will discuss in this chapter.

Stick to Unflavored Water, Coffee, or Tea

When following IF, it's important not to focus solely on the calories of the food you're eating and drinking, but more on the quality of what you are consuming. I mention this because when I started my What IF Diet journey, I first tried to find out what I could get away with during my fasts without breaking them. I thought that by allowing myself to keep my mouth busy or taste something pleasant, it would make fasting less painful. Unfortunately, I was wrong—very wrong. I figured as long as I stuck to calorie-free or artificially sweetened gum, tea, flavored water, etc., I could trick my body into thinking it was getting the food it craved so I could white-knuckle it until lunch. My biggest offender was diet soda. For the first few weeks of IF, I drank coffee with sugar-free creamer first thing in the morning, then diet soda until lunch, or whenever I decided to break my fast. Little did I know that drinking artificially sweetened beverages during my fasting window was only making it harder for me to push through the urge to eat.

Not realizing that this was the case, I decided to do a little research on how to keep myself "full" during a fast. I thought perhaps drinking more water would help, but...

Water, Water Everywhere... But All I Want is Diet Soda!

When I first started my What IF Diet Plan, there were days that I practically lived off coffee and diet soda and wouldn't have a sip of water all day. Diet soda was caffeinated, tasted good, and was cold and refreshing in the relentless South Texas heat. It gave me that get-up-and-go that I needed to get me through a long workday. Plus, it was sweet, so it kept me from craving food with real sugar. Or so I thought. Despite my love for diet soda, though, I knew water was the superior beverage and wanted to start drinking more of it.

To convince myself to do that, I decided to conduct some research on the topic. You see, I tend to overthink things, even things that seem common-sensical like "drink more water." If I'm going to implement something that I don't find pleasant into my life, I want to see evidence that it's worth doing. So I delved into my university's library to find research articles on hydration, dehydration, water and fat loss, water and hunger, etc. The surprising thing is, I didn't find many articles that supported my belief that I should be drinking more water. In fact, most of the articles I read didn't support the popular notion that drinking more water aids with fat loss or better health.

What Science Says About Drinking Water

One European study revealed that "lean young males" consumed fewer calories after drinking a pint of water immediately before eating, and therefore concluded that drinking water before meals could be a "good strategy" for suppressing caloric intake and managing weight.[26] It certainly sounded plausible. However, a closer look at this study made me second-guess the likelihood of that conclusion.

First of all, this study consisted of 14 lean young men who were *not* obese or needing to "manage" their weight. Plus, they were fed a *porridge breakfast* and remained in total isolation for 30 minutes while they ate. Well shoot! I would eat less too if I had to drink a pint of water, then eat porridge in total isolation. Just the thought of drinking water and eating porridge at seven o'clock in the morning makes me lose my appetite.

In contrast, a U.S. study found some mixed results when it came to using water to suppress hunger and calorie consumption.[27] In one experiment, results showed that drinking three 16-ounce bottles of water before lunch resulted in reduced calorie consumption at lunch for people considered "normal weight," but "had no effect on individuals categorized as overweight/obese." In an attempt to create a similar calorie reduction for the overweight subjects, researchers conducted a second experiment where the test subjects were made to drink *four 16-ounce bottles of water* before eating lunch. Yikes! In a surprising twist, the results of the second experiment revealed that there was *no difference* in the amount of calories consumed when compared to drinking no water before lunch.[27]

I found this study fascinating because the results replicated what might happen in real life. You see, in the second experiment with the four bottles of water, the subjects indeed *reported feeling less hungry*, but they still consumed the same number of calories as they did when they didn't chug water throughout the morning. This study was also truer to life because the test subjects were provided with a full lunch buffet, which consisted of pasta, Texas toast, fruit, and chocolate chip cookies, among other tasty items. Plus, there were no time restrictions on how long they had to eat, so they could take small breaks and go back for more food at their leisure.

These actions certainly sounded like normal human behavior. How many times before going to a party or buffet have you eaten something or drunk plenty of water to make sure you wouldn't be too hungry when the food arrives? Then, you still end up eating just as much as you would've normally. You may have even *believed* that you ate less, but that probably wasn't the case.

So how is it possible that filling up on a ton of water before eating doesn't reduce the amount of food or calories we eat? Well, as vital as water is to our overall health, it's not meant to trick our bodies into believing that we're less hungry. Plain water processes through the body pretty quickly and doesn't remain in the stomach long. Therefore, even if we drink a large amount of water right before a meal, chances are that it will keep us feeling full for a few minutes, but empty out by the time we've eaten half our meal. This results in feeling the same amount of hunger as we would have before drinking the water.

Furthermore, while rare, overhydration is a very real possibility for people who consume more water than necessary to satiate their thirst. An article published in the Physician and Sportsmedicine journal found that misinformation from the Internet regarding how much water we should drink when exercising can set people up for overhydration, which can cause sodium levels to drop fatally low.[28] This is especially noticeable in athletes who believe they need to drink more water or sports drinks to keep from getting dehydrated.[29]

The truth is, it is difficult for healthy adults living in a modern society to inadvertently become critically dehydrated. An experiment conducted in 2004 found that after 24 hours of restricting fluids, all test subjects reported an intense urge to drink something and "had to make a conscious effort" not to consume liquid for the sake of the experiment.[30] Researchers noted that the subjects of their study "would not have become dehydrated to this extent 'by accident.'"

All in all, water is an essential component for living, but more is not always better. Kidney specialist Dr. Mitchell Rosner, of the University of Virginia Health System, suggests that we listen to our bodies when it comes to determining how much water to drink. "If you drink when thirsty, you will not become hyponatremic, and you will not suffer from significant dehydration."[29] That's it! Easy, straightforward advice from an expert, and proof that we can keep our water worries at bay.

That still didn't resolve my whole issue, though. Sure, research shows that we don't need to drink gallons of water to lose weight and be healthy, but what did it say about diet soda and artificial sweeteners? Is drinking diet soda enough to keep us healthy and hydrated?

What Science Says about Diet Soda

In contrast to how I felt about my research on water, I was *not* pleasantly surprised with my findings on diet soda and artificial sweeteners. In fact, I was completely overwhelmed by the sheer volume of studies that linked diet soda to obesity and insulin resistance.

Several recent studies found that artificial and non-caloric sweeteners stimulate glucose intolerance by altering the gut's microbiome.[31, 32, 33] Numerous others found that higher consumption of artificial sweeteners was often linked to obesity and insulin resistance.[34-36] But the one I found most fascinating was a Mexican study published in April 2019 that found that *taking a single sip of an artificially sweetened beverage increased insulin levels in healthy adults.*[37]

This study randomly offered 45 healthy young test subjects a single sip (about two ounces) of plain water or artificially sweetened water, then tested their blood insulin and glucose levels at 15-minute intervals for two hours. As one would expect, the sip of water with artificial sweetener did not impact the test subjects' blood glucose levels.[37] After all, this is the main reason people with diabetes consume artificially sweetened products: the products should not raise their blood sugar.

However, the test subjects' *insulin* levels steadily increased over the course of two hours and were *doubled at the two-hour mark!*[37] Now, why should you care about increased insulin levels when fasting? Well, if you remember from my previous chapter, *The Power of Hormones*, insulin is a key player when it comes to hunger and fat storage. The higher your insulin levels are, the hungrier you will be, and less fat burning will take place.

Although IF offers many health benefits, I especially enjoy its effects on hunger. I like not feeling hungry throughout the day or worrying about what and when I will eat. However, by consuming artificial sweeteners during my fast, I was sabotaging those effects.

Drinking diet soda and other artificially sweetened indulgences during your fast is like playing "the boy who cried wolf" with your body. You're basically tricking your body into believing that it will receive food soon. In response, not only does your body release insulin to take care of the expected rise in blood sugar, but it also stops burning fat for fuel! After all, if your body is expecting fuel in the form of easily digestible calories (i.e., sugar), why should it waste more energy burning its own fat?

Although I'd heard of the pitfalls of drinking diet soda before, this last study really changed my perspective. I am convinced that drinking anything artificially flavored or sweetened induces false hunger signals and keeps the body from burning fat for fuel. If I drink an artificially sweetened beverage, I'll consume it as part of my meal or even as a treat before I close my eating window. I do not consume diet drinks anytime throughout my fasting window, and I highly recommend that you do the same if you want to reap the full benefits of IF and *The What IF? Diet Plan*.

Here is a list of items that can also trigger an insulin response if you consume them during your fast:

- Diet drinks of any kind

- Flavored waters

- Gum—sugar-free or regular

- Bullion powder or cubes (often have flavor enhancers, hidden sweeteners, etc.)

- Sugar-free syrups or creamers

- Pretty much any packaged product labeled "sugar-free" or "low-carb"

To simplify it further, keep away from anything tasty, sweet, or flavored while you are fasting. The whole point of fasting is that you are *not eating*. Trying to trick your body into believing it is receiving nourishment in the form of food when it's not derails the fasting process. As demonstrated by the previously referenced experiment, it takes only "one sip" or one taste of something sweet to increase insulin levels for several hours. This not only makes it harder to stick to your fast, but also shuts down the metabolic fat-burning process.

Be Prepa-a-a-ared!

I can't help but hear Uncle Scar's voice crooning out "Be prepa-a-a-ared!" in *The Lion King* as I'm writing this. In all seriousness though, there are a couple of reasons it pays to be prepared when fine-tuning your fasts. First, you may experience hunger pangs during the process of pushing your eating window back. This is normal since your body (and mind) may have been used to eating at certain times throughout the day. If your body was accustomed to getting a boost of energy from breakfast at 8 a.m., it won't be happy when you force it to wait until 10 a.m.

Plus, if you white-knuckle hunger pangs until your assigned eating time, you will most likely shove the first piece of food that you see into your mouth. This could be the meal that you planned to eat, or a candy bar from the vending machine, or leftover mac 'n' cheese from your toddler's plate (been there!). When your body is demanding caloric sustenance for energy, you shouldn't count on willpower to get you through.

The second reason you should be prepared when fine-tuning your fasts is that certain foods can *induce* hunger, rather than reduce it. In other words, you'll actually be hungrier after eating these types of foods than if you hadn't eaten anything at all. Foods that trigger large spikes in insulin are the foods that you want to avoid breaking your fast with. Instead, you can be prepared with *low-insulin-producing* snacks to tide you over until you're ready to eat a full meal.

As you may have guessed, foods that are high in sugar or refined carbohydrates will trigger higher spikes in insulin, and therefore hunger, than foods that are lower in refined carbohydrates. However, even foods that are low in carbohydrates but artificially flavored or sweetened (such as low-carb protein bars) can also spike insulin and make you hungrier. Therefore, it's best to have plain or savory, unsweetened, low-carb snacks on hand in preparation for breaking your fast.

Here is a list of some of the best items I've found for breaking a fast:

- All-natural bone broth—homemade or store bought

- Canned or pouched tuna—preferably plain, but flavored works too

- Pork rinds—preferably plain, but flavored is OK

- 1-2 handfuls of macadamia nuts—plain or salted

- Boiled eggs

- Unsweetened beef or turkey jerky

- 1-3 strips of bacon

- 1-2 ounces of plain cream cheese

If you're thinking this list of items sounds bland, or not all that appetizing, you're right. When breaking your fasts, it's helpful to consume foods that are nourishing, not necessarily tasty. These foods will keep your insulin levels low, and help you learn to identify *true* hunger from conditioned hunger.

So if you're feeling hunger pangs at 10 a.m., but are not scheduled to eat until 11 a.m., ask yourself if you're hungry enough to eat one of these low-insulin-producing foods. If the answer is no, then you're probably feeling conditioned hunger pangs because it's "about that time" to eat.

If you have less than an hour until you break your fast, try asking yourself the personalized "What IF" questions you wrote down previously, and see if you can push through that hour *10 minutes at a time*. If the hunger pangs are causing you to feel miserable, overly distracted, or irritable, then break your fast early with one of the low insulin producing snacks or meals listed above. You will satisfy your hunger and keep your body burning fat for fuel.

Feeling Hungry? Take a Nap!

Believe it or not, getting adequate sleep is vital to fine-tuning your fasts. Not getting enough sleep leads to haphazard hunger cues throughout the day and makes it much more difficult to stick to your fasting window. I believe this occurs because although the body craves sleep, it's not always possible to take a nap during the day. When we force the body to stay awake, it signals our brain that we need fuel to stay awake and function properly. The easiest, fastest form of fuel we can give our body is food.

It took me a while to figure out that getting inadequate sleep was sabotaging my fasting efforts. Often, I'd come home voracious for dinner, even if I'd already eaten a couple of hours earlier. I'd scarf down my meal without even tasting it, then sit down to relax and immediately fall asleep. Unfortunately, I'd often wake up around 10 at night, have trouble falling back asleep, stay up all night, then start the cycle all over the next day.

At first I thought IF was disrupting my sleep cycle, and I've indeed heard anecdotal stories about this occurring. But by analyzing my situation and asking myself some helpful "What IF?" questions, I soon figured out that my insufficient sleep was throwing off my body's hunger signals. To test my theory, I forced myself to lie down and take a short nap one afternoon as soon as I got home from work. My brain and stomach rebelled and urged me to grab a small snack first, or just see what was in the fridge, or help the kids with homework, but I ignored my internal tantrum and lay in bed with my eyes closed until I fell asleep.

When I woke up an hour later, I felt refreshed and my hunger had completely subsided! I got up, made dinner, ate normally and consciously, then went about the rest of my evening. I could not believe how interconnected my sleep was with my hunger!

Now, I know it's not always possible to get adequate sleep at night or take a nap during the day. As a mother of three boys and a former nightshift worker, I know that sleep can be an elusive luxury. The first few years of your child's life means little to no sleep for you. Newborn babies take all your time and energy, leaving little time for yourself or sleep. As they get older, sleep is easier to come by, but it can take years to get back to a normal sleeping pattern—if you even had one in the first place. Of course, being sleep-deprived is only one of many stressors that motherhood can bring. Add to that post-partum issues, never having time to yourself, being isolated from friends, and constantly serving meals and snacks to your little one, and it's no wonder losing baby weight can be so difficult!

When I worked overnights as a fast-food manager, I constantly craved sweets throughout my shift. Instead of drinking black coffee, I began adding a ton of flavored creamer to my coffee—and it was never enough! Eventually, I began making my own mock Frappuccinos by adding some vanilla shake into my coffee instead. As a result, my waistline increased exponentially during the first few months of working overnights. Fortunately, I was able to find a good day job soon after and got back into a normal sleep routine.

Therefore, while I realize the struggles related to getting adequate sleep, it's worth being cognizant of the need for it. If you find yourself having cravings or feeling more hungry than usual, stop and assess whether you've been getting enough sleep. If you know you haven't, try to see where you can make small improvements in your sleep patterns. You also may need to ask yourself some "What IF?" questions if you believe that getting enough sleep at night or taking a nap is not a possibility. Here is a list of the "What IF?" questions I asked myself when I decided to make sleep a priority in my life:

What IF my body is craving sleep, not food?

What IF I don't have to help the boys with homework today?

What IF getting a nap in is worth missing football practice?

What IF putting myself first is setting a good example for my kids?

What IF my husband can handle the bedtime routine tonight so I can get to sleep at a decent hour?

Once I asked myself these "What IF?" questions, it became easier to make sleep a priority and opened me up to new opportunities I would've never thought of. For example, when I decided that I would skip taking my boys to football practice so I could get some rest, I messaged their team to let them know we couldn't make it. Unexpectedly, one of the parents quickly messaged me back and offered to take my boys to practice so they wouldn't miss out.

I was immediately wracked with guilt about the offer because I felt that my reason for not taking them to practice was not a good one. Sure I was tired, but what parent isn't? The parent called and said he and his wife insisted on picking up the boys for me. He assured me that there was plenty of room in their SUV, and that his son loved playing with my boys. I timidly took their kind offer and stayed home and relaxed while my kids went to practice. After practice, the parents messaged me to let me know that they were taking the boys out to eat too. I was stunned and beyond grateful!

Had I not taken the time to recognize that my body needed sleep and asked myself those helpful "What IF?" questions, I would have ended up taking my kids to practice, been irritable the entire time, then come home and probably binged on junk food to quell my misery. By choosing to identify what my body really needed and making myself a priority, I was able to get the rest I needed, *and* my boys were able to make it to football practice, then have a great time eating dinner with their friend and teammate. Plus, my husband and I are still friends with these incredible parents to this day.

A Full Day of Fasting

My last tip for fine-tuning your fasting is to try a full day of fasting, if possible. At this phase in the plan, I hope that you have been practicing IF consistently for several weeks and that you're feeling good and witnessing some great results. Perhaps you've lost a few inches or are feeling less tired and achy. Maybe you've had more mental clarity and stamina to get through your day. If so, that's excellent news!

If you've been consistent with your fasting/eating windows and experienced some of the benefits, you may want to try a full day of fasting, which means going at least 24 hours without food. Now this might sound like a total nightmare to fellow foodies, but I promise that it's not nearly as difficult as it sounds. In fact, the first time I fasted for 24 hours was simply another "What IF?" moment for me.

As mentioned previously, I am full-time employee and part-time graduate student, as well as a wife and mother. My schedule is quite full, as you can imagine. One Sunday, I was working on a research paper for school that was due by midnight. I woke up, got the kids fed and settled, then got straight to writing and completing my assignment.

My husband got home from his job around 2 p.m., so I took a break from writing to spend time with the family and make an early dinner. We finished eating around five, and I went back to focusing on my paper until it was completed around eight at night. I closed my laptop in relief and went straight to the kitchen to grab a snack and a well-deserved glass of wine. However, I quickly realized that I wasn't even hungry. I thought, *Why eat if I'm not hungry?*

Of course my brain came up with a million reasons why I should eat something:

You still have two hours left in your eating window!

After finishing that assignment, you deserve a snack!

It's the weekend… live a little!

You know your husband will want you to eat with him.

If you don't eat now, you will be starving *by tomorrow!*

Fortunately, at this point in my What IF Diet Plan, I knew better than to listen to these frenetic thoughts. I had proven my old beliefs about food and hunger wrong in the past, so who was to say these beliefs weren't wrong too? Instead, I asked myself:

What IF I didn't eat just because I have "time" to eat?

What IF I rewarded myself with something other than food?

What IF I didn't use weekends as an excuse to eat more?

What IF I didn't eat just because the family is eating?

What IF I'm not starving *by tomorrow?*

What IF my body can benefit from a longer fast?

At that moment, I decided that I was not going to eat just because I had time left in my eating window. I'd finished eating by 5 p.m. that day and would see if I could "survive" without food until 5 p.m. the next day. At this point in the plan, it didn't even seem like that big a deal. And you know what? It wasn't.

The next day was a Monday, so family, work, and school kept me busy as always. If I was any hungrier than usual that day, it wasn't memorable, or anything that would deter me from pursuing future full-day fasts. When 5 p.m. rolled around, I opened my eating window with some bone broth, then ate as I would any other day. I was proud of myself for continuing to challenge my old beliefs and way of thinking.

Fasting for 24 hours or more is not always necessary for losing weight. If you've been losing weight with your current fasting windows, and you're not interested in reaping the other benefits of fasting, then more power to you! After all, *The What IF? Diet Plan* was created and written to fit your lifestyle… not to make life more complicated.

Still, there are a myriad of benefits to fasting for a full day. Research shows that after 24 hours of fasting, the body generates 70% of its energy from the process of gluconeogenesis.[38] This means the body produces energy from excess glucose that is stored in our fat and muscle. In fact, partaking in full-day fasts intermittently for several weeks has proven effective in reducing body fat, total cholesterol levels, and triglycerides in normal weight and obese individuals.[39]

A study from the University of Cambridge also found that levels of growth hormone naturally increased in both men and women after 24 hours of fasting.[40] Growth hormone is an important regulator in fat and carbohydrate metabolism, as well as muscle growth and repair.

Other studies found that fasting for 24 hours can reduce risk factors for heart disease.[41]

Personally, I enjoy doing a 24-hour fast at least once a month, usually the week after my monthly cycle. I find it rejuvenating and feel that it allows my body to naturally reset. I wake up the next day feeling energetic, less bloated, and ready to open my window with nourishing foods. Plus, many people find that fasting for 24 hours is a great way to restart weight loss if they've hit a plateau. If you feel ready to take the plunge, try it and see how you feel.

AFTERWORD

Whoo hoo! I am so happy that you've made it to the end of *The What IF? Diet Plan*! I hope that you've been able to implement the phases of the plan into your daily life, and that you are asking yourself positive "What IF?" questions to help reveal new possibilities for you to consider. By asking yourself "What IF?" and pushing past the boundaries of your old beliefs, you will discover that you can accomplish incredible feats you never knew you were capable of. I encourage you to practice writing useful "What IF?" questions anytime you come up against an obstacle in your life or begin doubting your ability to change. I have provided some pages at the end of this section so you can get started.

Also, remember to congratulate yourself on any and all accomplishments that you've made over these past few weeks or months. If you've lost inches, lessened cravings, reduced inflammation, gained mental clarity, or stuck to your new eating/fasting windows consistently, then give yourself a round of applause. Keep in mind that the small everyday wins are what keep you on the road to victory.

Finally, if you found the information in this book helpful, please be sure to spread the word to your friends and family. You can also leave a positive review on Amazon to help others discover the plan too. If you ever have any questions about following the

plan, or simply need a word of encouragement, please feel free to follow my blog at:
www.thewhatifdietplan.com or email me at:
alexis@thewhatifdietplan.com. Please know that you truly have the power to change your life, and by doing so you also serve as a beacon of hope to everyone around you!

What IF

_____

_____ ?

What IF

_____

_____ ?

What IF

_____

_____ ?

What IF

_____

_____ ?

What IF

_____

_____ ?

THE WHAT IF? DIET PLAN

What IF

_____

_____?

What IF

_____

_____?

What IF

_____

_____?

What IF

_____

_____?

What IF

_____

_____?

What IF

_____

_____?

What IF

_____

_____?

What IF

_____
_____ ?

What IF

_____
_____ ?

What IF

_____
_____ ?

What IF

_____
_____ ?

What IF

_____
_____ ?

What IF

_____
_____ ?

What IF

_____
_____ ?

THE WHAT IF? DIET PLAN

What IF

_____
_____ ?

What IF

_____
_____ ?

What IF

_____
_____ ?

What IF

_____
_____ ?

What IF

_____
_____ ?

What IF

_____
_____ ?

What IF

_____
_____ ?

REFERENCES

1. Byrne, N., Sainsbury, A., King, N. et al. Intermittent energy restriction improves weight loss efficiency in obese men: the MATADOR study. *Int J Obes* 42, 129–138 (2018). https://doi.org/10.1038/ijo.2017.206

2. Moro T, Tinsley G, Bianco A, et al. Effects of eight weeks of time-restricted feeding (16/8) on basal metabolism, maximal strength, body composition, inflammation, and cardiovascular risk factors in resistance-trained males. *J Transl Med*. 2016;14(1):290. Published 2016 Oct 13. doi:10.1186/s12967-016-1044-0

3. Tinsley GM, Forsse JS, Butler NK, et al. Time-restricted feeding in young men performing resistance training: A randomized controlled trial. *Eur J Sport Sci*. 2017;17(2):200-207. doi:10.1080/17461391.2016.1223173

4. Catenacci VA, Pan Z, Ostendorf D, et al. A randomized pilot study comparing zero-calorie alternate-day fasting to daily caloric restriction in adults with obesity. *Obesity (Silver Spring)*. 2016;24(9):1874-1883. doi:10.1002/oby.21581

5. Zenoozi, ZMZ, Ali Noori, SM. Association of fasting with heavy metals and minerals. *Journal of Fasting and Health*. 2017;5(4):158-161. DOI 10.22038/jfh.2018.29603.1109

6. Mendelsohn AR, Larrick JW. Prolonged fasting/refeeding promotes hematopoietic stem cell regeneration and

rejuvenation. *Rejuvenation Res*. 2014;17(4):385-389. doi:10.1089/rej.2014.1595

7. Cheng CW, Adams GB, Perin L, et al. Prolonged fasting reduces IGF-1/PKA to promote hematopoietic-stem-cell-based regeneration and reverse immunosuppression [published correction appears in Cell Stem Cell. 2016 Feb 4;18(2):291-2]. *Cell Stem Cell*. 2014;14(6):810-823. doi:10.1016/j.stem.2014.04.014

8. Milne, S., Orbell, S. and Sheeran, P. (2002), Combining motivational and volitional interventions to promote exercise participation: Protection motivation theory and implementation intentions. *British Journal of Health Psychology*, 7: 163-184. doi:10.1348/135910702169420

9. Fothergill, E., Guo, J., Howard, L., Kerns, J.C., Knuth, N.D., Brychta, R., Chen, K.Y., Skarulis, M.C., Walter, M., Walter, P.J. and Hall, K.D. (2016), Persistent metabolic adaptation 6 years after "The Biggest Loser" competition. *Obesity*, 24: 1612-1619. doi:10.1002/oby.21538

10. Kolata, G., After "The Biggest Loser," their bodies fought to regain the weight. The New York Times. https://www.nytimes.com/2016/05/02/health/biggest-loser-weight-loss.html. Published May 2016.

11. Kerns, J.C., Guo, J., Fothergill, E., Howard, L., Knuth, N.D., Brychta, R., Chen, K.Y., Skarulis, M.C., Walter, P.J. and Hall, K.D. (2017), Increased Physical Activity Associated with Less Weight

REFERENCES

Regain Six Years After "The Biggest Loser" Competition. *Obesity*, 25: 1838-1843. doi:10.1002/oby.21986

12. Sáinz N, Barrenetxe J, Moreno-Aliaga MJ, Martínez JA. Leptin resistance and diet-induced obesity: central and peripheral actions of leptin. *Metabolism*. https://www.sciencedirect.com/science/article/pii/S0026049514003096. Published October 23, 2014.

13. Mattson MP, Longo VD, Harvie M. Impact of intermittent fasting on health and disease processes. *Ageing Research Reviews*. https://www.sciencedirect.com/science/article/pii/S1568163716302513. Published October 31, 2016.

14. Hoddy KK, Gibbons C, Kroeger CM, et al. Changes in hunger and fullness in relation to gut peptides before and after 8 weeks of alternate day fasting. *Clinical Nutrition*. https://www.sciencedirect.com/science/article/pii/S0261561416001023. Published March 30, 2016.

15. Taheri S, Lin L, Austin D, Young T, Mignot E. Short sleep duration is associated with reduced leptin, elevated ghrelin, and increased body mass index. *PLoS Med*. 2004;1(3):e62. doi:10.1371/journal.pmed.0010062

16. Spiegel K, Tasali E, Penev P, Van Cauter E. Brief communication: Sleep curtailment in healthy young men is associated with decreased leptin levels, elevated ghrelin levels, and increased hunger and appetite. *Ann Intern Med*.

2004;141(11):846-850. doi:10.7326/0003-4819-141-11-200412070-00008

17. Sinha R, Gu P, Hart R, Guarnaccia JB. Food craving, cortisol and ghrelin responses in modeling highly palatable snack intake in the laboratory. *Physiology & Behavior*. https://www.sciencedirect.com/science/article/pii/S0031938419301179. Published May 27, 2019.

18. Leidy HJ, Gardner JK, Frye BR, et al. Circulating ghrelin is sensitive to changes in body weight during a diet and exercise program in normal-weight young women. *J Clin Endocrinol Metab*. 2004;89(6):2659-2664. doi:10.1210/jc.2003-031471

19. Mason, C., Xiao, L., Imayama, I., Duggan, C.R., Campbell, K.L., Kong, A., Wang, C.-Y., Alfano, C.M., Blackburn, G.L., Foster-Schubert, K.E. and McTiernan, A. (2015), The effects of separate and combined dietary weight loss and exercise on fasting ghrelin concentrations in overweight and obese women: a randomized controlled trial. *Clin Endocrinol*, 82: 369-376. doi:10.1111/cen.12483

20. Druce MR, Wren AM, Park AJ, et al. Ghrelin increases food intake in obese as well as lean subjects. *Int J Obes (Lond)*. 2005;29(9):1130-1136. doi:10.1038/sj.ijo.0803001

21. Alzoghaibi MA, Pandi-Perumal SR, Sharif MM, BaHammam AS (2014) Diurnal Intermittent Fasting during Ramadan: The Effects on Leptin and Ghrelin Levels. *PLoS ONE* 9(3): e92214. https://doi.org/10.1371/journal.pone.0092214

REFERENCES

22. Natalucci, G, Riedl, S, Gleiss, A, Zidek, T, & Frisch, H. (2005). Spontaneous 24-h ghrelin secretion pattern in fasting subjects: maintenance of a meal-related pattern, *European Journal of Endocrinology eur j endocrinol*, 152(6), 845-850.

23. Praag Hvan, Fleshner M, Schwartz MW, Mattson MP. Exercise, Energy Intake, Glucose Homeostasis, and the Brain. *Journal of Neuroscience.* https://www.jneurosci.org/content/34/46/15139. Published November 12, 2014.

24. Longo VD, Mattson MP. Fasting: molecular mechanisms and clinical applications. *Cell Metab*. 2014;19(2):181-192. doi:10.1016/j.cmet.2013.12.008

25. Chamari K, Briki W, Farooq A, Patrick T, Belfekih T, Herrera CP. Impact of Ramadan intermittent fasting on cognitive function in trained cyclists: a pilot study. *Biol Sport*. 2016;33(1):49-56. doi:10.5604/20831862.1185888

26. Corney, R.A., Sunderland, C. & James, L.J. Immediate pre-meal water ingestion decreases voluntary food intake in lean young males. *Eur J Nutr* 55, 815–819 (2016). https://doi.org/10.1007/s00394-015-0903-4

27. McKay NJ, Belous IV, Temple JL. Increasing water intake influences hunger and food preference, but does not reliably suppress energy intake in adults. *Physiology & Behavior.* https://www.sciencedirect.com/science/article/abs/pii/S0031938418302051. Published April 17, 2018.

28. Martin D. Hoffman, Theodore L. Bross III & R. Tyler Hamilton (2016) Are we being drowned by overhydration advice on the Internet?, *The Physician and Sportsmedicine*, 44:4, 343-348, DOI: 10.1080/00913847.2016.1222853

29. Swensen E. Experts: Overhydration Potentially Deadly for Athletes. *UVA Today*. https://news.virginia.edu/content/experts-overhydration-potentially-deadly-athletes. Published October 19, 2018.

30. Shirreffs SM, Merson SJ, Fraser SM, Archer DT. The effects of fluid restriction on hydration status and subjective feelings in man. *British Journal of Nutrition*. 2004;91(6):951-958. doi:10.1079/BJN20041149

31. Suez, J., Korem, T., Zeevi, D. *et al.* Artificial sweeteners induce glucose intolerance by altering the gut microbiota. *Nature* 514, 181–186 (2014). https://doi.org/10.1038/nature13793

32. Nettleton JE, Reimer RA, Shearer J. Reshaping the gut microbiota: Impact of low calorie sweeteners and the link to insulin resistance? *Physiology & Behavior*. https://www.sciencedirect.com/science/article/pii/S0031938416301640. Published April 15, 2016.

33. Abdelhadi J, Simone D, King CH, Mazumder R, Crandall KA, Sylvetsky-Meni AC. Effects of three-times daily diet soda consumption for one week on the composition of the gut microbiome in healthy young adults. *Health Sciences Research Commons*.

REFERENCES

https://hsrc.himmelfarb.gwu.edu/gw_research_days/2016/GW SPH_Marvin/56/.

34. Fowler, S.P., Williams, K., Resendez, R.G., Hunt, K.J., Hazuda, H.P. and Stern, M.P. (2008), Fueling the Obesity Epidemic? Artificially Sweetened Beverage Use and Long-term Weight Gain. *Obesity*, 16: 1894-1900. doi:10.1038/oby.2008.284

35. Shearer J, Nettleton J. Artificially sweetened taste of insulin resistance?. *Appl Physiol Nutr Metab*. 2016;41(7):iii. doi:10.1139/apnm-2016-0294

36. Green E, Murphy C. Altered processing of sweet taste in the brain of diet soda drinkers. *Physiology & Behavior*. https://www.ncbi.nlm.nih.gov/pubmed/22583859. Published November 5, 2012.

37. Angélica Y. Gómez-Arauz, Nallely Bueno-Hernández, Leon F. Palomera, Raúl Alcántara-Suárez, Karen L. De León, Lucía A. Méndez-García, Miguel Carrero-Aguirre, Aaron N. Manjarrez-Reyna, Camilo P. Martínez-Reyes, Marcela Esquivel-Velázquez, Alejandra Ruiz-Barranco, Neyla Baltazar-López, Sergio Islas-Andrade, Galileo Escobedo, Guillermo Meléndez, A single 48 mg sucralose sip unbalances monocyte subpopulations and stimulates insulin secretion in healthy young adults, *Journal of Immunology Research*, vol. 2019, Article ID 6105059, 10 pages, 2019. https://doi.org/10.1155/2019/6105059

38. Katz J, Medicine 1 Dof I, Tayek JA, et al. Gluconeogenesis and the Cori cycle in 12-, 20-, and 40-h-fasted humans. American Journal of Physiology-Endocrinology and Metabolism.

https://journals.physiology.org/doi/full/10.1152/ajpendo.1998.275.3.e537. Published September 1, 1998.

39. Grant M. Tinsley, Paul M. La Bounty, Effects of intermittent fasting on body composition and clinical health markers in humans, *Nutrition Reviews*, Volume 73, Issue 10, October 2015, Pages 661–674, https://doi.org/10.1093/nutrit/nuv041

40. Salgin B, Marcovecchio ML, Hill N, Dunger DB, Frystyk J. The effect of prolonged fasting on levels of growth hormone-binding protein and free growth hormone. *Growth Horm IGF Res*. 2012;22(2):76-81. doi:10.1016/j.ghir.2012.02.003

41. Horne BD, Benjamin D Horne Search for more papers by this author, Cox JE, et al. Abstract 13412: 24-Hour Water-Only Fasting Acutely Reduces Trimethylamine N-Oxide: the FEELGOOD Trial. Circulation. https://www.ahajournals.org/doi/abs/10.1161/circ.130.suppl_2.13412. Published March 27, 2018.

CPSIA information can be obtained
at www.ICGtesting.com
Printed in the USA
BVHW031437140622
639735BV00016B/1292